ANIMAL RESCUE

ANIMAL RESCUE

VALERIE PORTER

In consultation with
the RSPCA Wildlife Department

ASHFORD
Southampton

Published by Ashford
          1 Church Road
          Shedfield
          Hampshire
          SO3 2HW

British Library Cataloguing in Publication Data

Porter, Valerie, *1942—*
  Animal rescue.
  1. Animals. Injuries. Emergency treatment
  I. Title
  636.089'71026

  ISBN 1-85253-196-7

Illustrations by Dave Stephens
Typeset by Staples Printers Rochester Limited, Love Lane, Rochester, Kent.
Printed by Hartnolls Limited, Bodmin, Cornwall, England.

CONTENTS

11. THE RESCUERS

LIST OF FIGURES

ACKNOWLEDGEMENTS

Many, many people have helped me with this book and my gratitude to them all is immeasurable. In particular I should like to thank the following: Eric and Eileen Ashby, and their foxes and badgers; Michael Bignold, BORIS; Ian and Valerie Brice, Pinewood Owl Parliament; Molly Burkett, Animal Rehabilitation Centre; Maurice Burton; Cats Protection League; Gay and Andrew Christie, Hessilhead Wildlife Rescue; John Cooper, Royal College of Surgeons; Lynn Cornick, Hydestile; John Cripps, on birds of prey; Grahame Dangerfield and Caroline Brown; Roger Ewbank, UFAW; Dennis Fenter, Brent Lodge, and his team; John Goodman, Mallydams Sanctuary and Field Centre; Jim Green, Vincent Wildlife Trust; Bill Jordan, Care for the Wild; Margaret King, Bird Rescue Association; James K. Kirkwood, Zoological Society of London; Laurance J. Larmour, Sea Life Centre, Oban; National Animal Rescue Association; Harold Nickerson, Marine Life Rescue; Jim Sargent, Norfolk Owl Rescue; Carol Scott, on birds of prey and other insights; Colin Seddon, Little Creech RSPCA Wildlife Unit; Bob Stebbings, ITE; Les Stocker, and his hedgehogs; Swan Rescue Service, Norfolk; Tim Thomas, RSPCA Wildlife Officer; Joanna Vinson, Birds of Prey Rescue Centre; Eileen Watkinson, Three Owls Bird Sanctuary; John Whitaker, MRCVS, BVMS.

INTRODUCTION

WHY CARE?

As these are, so am I.
Sutta Nipata

It is said that the British never really grow up and that this is why they are animal lovers. All over the world animals are exploited and abused, either deliberately or through ignorance, carelessness and disinterest, but it seems to be the British more than any other nationality (except perhaps the Americans and Dutch) who care for garden birds, worry about endangered species, surround themselves with pets, abhor cruelty to animals, object to battery-hen systems and veal-calf crates, and support sanctuaries, hospitals, rest-homes, rescue centres, welfare groups and trusts for wild and domestic-ated lost, hurt, abandoned or maltreated creatures.

Horses and donkeys, dogs, cats, wild birds, foxes and hedgehogs seem to be the most popular beneficiaries of this great fund of goodwill; more recently the stranded or sick mammals of the oceans have become subjects of the kind of human concern and co-ordinated action that has brought nations together in huge rescue operations which only the most die-hard cynic could suggest were for less than altruistic motives.

What is it about distressed animals that seems to generate as much compassion (and sometimes more) in the human heart as for distressed people? Why do we go to such lengths to rescue a living creature, regardless of whether or not its species is "attractive" or abundant? Why do people risk their own lives for drowning dogs, trapped cats, livestock in burning buildings, wild creatures suffering from the effects of man-made pollution or being massacred by poachers or traffic? Why do we empty our pockets to help wild-bird hospitals and rest-homes for horses? Why do we care?

Many people have begun to realise how the urban races are increasingly cutting themselves off from the rest of the living world, a world of which human beings have always been an integral part but where now there is too little room for animals other than the human ones who have constructed for themselves—willingly, it seems—largely artificial environments.

1

But we, too, are animals and we need the company of other animals. Our compassion embraces them and animals keep faith with us. Even in the cities and the suburbs, animals live amongst us—domestic pets and strays, urban foxes and badgers, garden-raiding deer and hedgehogs, and of course all kinds of birds, rodents and insects. Bats live in the snug attics of housing estates; toads and frogs continue to visit their ancestral breeding places even if they are now at the heart of a new town.

Yet as a civilisation we are more often causative in bringing distress to other animals than in relieving it. Our cars are responsible for countless deaths and injuries on the roads; our pollution destroys the environment for vast numbers of creatures, poisons their internal systems, or entraps them, drowns them, burns them, covers them with oil. Our material greed eradicates their habitats and we seem to be galloping towards a future where the only living creatures will be humans and the domesticated animals who serve our needs. What an appalling arrogance!

Perhaps it is in reaction to this relentlessly deepening chasm between mankind and the rest of the living world that some people—more and more of us—reach out to take up an injured bird, give shelter to a sportsman's prey or offer a home to an abused or abandoned dog. It is an attempt to redress the balance and to counter the unwitting inhumanity of man, to remain part of the whole living world, not apart from it.

Because there are so many animal casualties (and throughout this book the term "animal" naturally includes birds) and because there is an inclination to help them, anyone who is known to have successfully rescued a casualty will soon be overwhelmed with injured, orphaned and abandoned creatures brought in by the general public. One of the aims of this book is to suggest what you can do yourself to ease an animal's distress immediately. But you will also need to take a more long-term view, right from the moment an animal comes into your care, and you thereby assume responsibility for its future welfare. With wild creatures in particular, it is never merely a case of easing physical pain or even of saving a life. The aim of every rescuer of wildlife, whether the victim is a sparrow or a sparrowhawk, a woodmouse or a deer, should be to prepare the animal adequately for a successful return to its natural lifestyle—in the wild. This act of rehabilitation is far more difficult—and controversial—than the initial act of rescue and nursing care, and part of this book is devoted to it.

Many a well-meaning person has caused more harm than good to the creatures they have tried to help, and sometimes their motives may not have been quite as generous as they believed. There is considerable satisfaction to be gained from caring for a distressed and dependent creature (human or otherwise) but personal gratification and a glowing sense of achievement might sometimes mean more than the creature's real welfare. It is flattering when a wild animal learns to trust you, but is it really in its best interests? If it trusts you, it might also trust other humans—and that could be fatal.

And we are selective, it must be admitted. Those who would devote time, funds and love to the care of fledglings or donkeys might not think twice about swatting a wasp, setting a mousetrap, or eradicating garden moles. Some say that the sign of a truly caring wildlife rescue centre is that pigeons, starlings and sparrows are as welcome as owls and swallows, that sanctuary is as readily given to toads and housemice as to endearing fox cubs. Others would argue that to rescue members of locally abundant species is to interfere with the local ecological balance. With domesticated species the arguments are different but none the less passionate, and indeed the whole world of animal rescue fairly bristles with opinions, beliefs and prejudice. One of the major debating points is whether or not any of us can assume the right to "play God" with the life of an animal, and this is a subject which each person must consider privately to decide whether their motives are as sound as their abilities to care for that animal.

There are probably thousands of people in this country quietly getting on with the job of caring for animal casualties, some with help from the general public but almost all without help from the State. For the inexperienced person who comes across a casualty of any kind it is very often better to go straight to the specialists for help rather than causing additional stress to the animal because of their own mishandling or ignorance. This book therefore includes not only advice on what you might call "do-it-yourself rescue" but also a section on where to go for expert help and advice or where to take a casualty you are unable or unwilling to care for yourself.

The directory of rescue organisations in Chapter 11 is not comprehensive, since every neighbourhood will have its own rescue groups and individuals with experience of casualties, but it does attempt to include some of the better-established and more respected centres, or those that specialise in a particular species. However, the inclusion of a centre in the directory does not necessarily imply personal recommendation nor does exclusion imply a lack of faith. Many of them are already overwhelmed by the numbers brought to them for care and have pleaded not to be included: they are already well enough known locally without attracting more candidates for their attention, though they will never turn away an animal in distress. Others have asked that only an indication of their whereabouts should be given, partly because their capacities are already overstretched and partly because members of the public who find a casualty are frequently insensitive to the resources, both human and financial, which are involved in animal rescue, and may even be critical if the centre's efforts are not successful.

Many of the people I have met who are engaged in rescue think nothing of sleepless nights, decades without so much as a week's holiday, constant concern over what might seem the most insignificant of animal lives—and all for no more than the desire to alleviate an animal's distress. How many of us are good enough to do the same?

One final point: exchanging information and the pooling of knowledge are in the interests of the animals. To do this, it is helpful if as many people as possible—from those who care for one little fledgling in the kitchen to those who take in hundreds of casualties every year—keep detailed records of their work and publish them in order to broadcast their experiences. We all learn from experience, be it our own or other people's, and one of the great advantages of being human is that we can communicate in words to thousands—millions—of other people. The person who keeps exotic animals and the person who looks after humble wildlife can find a great deal in common; each can share their techniques to the benefit of the other. Those who breed from captive common species can pass on their knowledge to those who are trying to breed a species close to extinction. If everyone who is interested in animal rescue contributes to the pool of knowledge, the quality of life will be successfully restored to many more animals; and if all those people quietly spread the word about the need to respect other animals, then perhaps, gradually, they can begin to open the eyes of those who ignore, exploit or directly abuse the world we all share.

CHAPTER ONE

ANIMALS IN DISTRESS

CARE

Squashed corpses are so common on our roads that they are no more than part of the scenery, almost as accepted as white lines, cat's-eyes and other highway furniture. Most of them are squirrels, hedgehogs and rabbits, though sometimes the coat colour of a flattened mess of meat betrays a dead fox or badger, or perhaps a cat or dog. In certain areas deer are the victims, their size being such that drivers cannot fail to be aware of the mutual impact, though deer are more often injured than killed. In some places at the appropriate season the shapes that seem to be dead leaves moving in the wind are in reality hosts of migrating amphibians, whose ancestors knew nothing of tarmac and speeding vehicles when they established their traditional breeding ponds. Sometimes there are birds—unwary fledglings, newly released pheasants who are not yet streetwise, parent birds playing "chicken" in the urgent spring search for nestling food, or owls dazzled by headlights, which seem to mesmerise so many creatures.

Usually the victims are killed on impact, or at least by the following vehicle. But sometimes—and more often than is realised—they are only injured: stunned, perhaps, or with a smashed limb or wing, or ruptured internal organs, or paralysed by a broken spine. Few drivers notice these victims, especially at night when the toll is highest, and fewer still will actually stop to help.

The desire to help should not be discouraged but the gesture should be tempered with caution, whether the motivation is pure compassion or even guilt at the distress the human race can cause as it rushes along. An empathy with animals is the natural precursor to the urge to help them but it needs to be exercised objectively and with a real understanding of the animal's immediate and long-term needs.

It is on the roads, perhaps, that most people encounter wildlife casualties but there are many other man-made situations that can unwittingly cause distress. Deer become trapped in snares set for foxes and rabbits; birds become entangled in gardeners' nylon mesh; swans collide with power lines or ingest old lead fishing weights; flocks of birds lose the argument with jet engines; sparrowhawks fly headlong into windows; ducks used to eating bread cast on the waters swallow a baited and barbed fishing line; fawns have their limbs severed and leverets are cut to shreds by the blades of the haycutter; tiny young toads and froglets are massacred by garden mowers; badgers are electrocuted on newly charged railway lines; seabirds are encased in oil; untold numbers of unknown creatures die unpleasantly from incidental poisoning or are sickened or born deformed by environmental pollution.

These are the accidental casualties of man's abuse of the environment. Then there are the more deliberate victims of hunters, coursers, baiters, tormentors and vandals. There are huge numbers of casualties from domestic cat predation and some from savaging by domestic dogs. There are many more "natural" casualties, of course—the victims of wild native predators, lightning strikes, territorial battles, over-population, epidemics, genetic weakness, violent storms, floods, heathland fires, harsh winters, and apparently inexplicable phenomena like mass beachings of stranded whales.

Then there are the abandoned young: the cubs of a snared vixen or badger sow killed by traffic, the nestlings deprived of a parent by a hungry hawk, hunting cat or airgun pellet, the ducklings left unbrooded and chilled because a fox or a shooter took their mother. In the wild, without human interference, a proportion of such tragedies is part of the delicate ecological balancing act, but human activities, especially of more recent years, have tipped that balance alarmingly to the detriment of wildlife, and it is therefore humans who must redress it.

At this point, please heed a firm warning. Many apparently abandoned young creatures are not in fact abandoned—but they soon will be if you interfere. These little ones are at a disadvantage immediately a human being steps in to "help", and thousands of them are thus put at risk by well-meaning people who think they are helping but who are in fact unwittingly signing death warrants on young lives. In late spring the rescue centres are inundated with such creatures—fledglings, fawns, cubs and leverets in particular—which are in fact victims of human ignorance rather than of parental neglect. If you come across a youngster, **leave it alone.** Do not jump to the conclusion that it needs assistance, unless it is quite clearly injured, trapped or in danger from predators. Retreat discreetly, and watch from a distance. It is more than likely that the parents are well aware of its whereabouts and welfare and they will return in their own good time to resume their duties, with a far greater chance of rearing their young successfully than you have.

Of course your heart goes out to a helpless fledgling or cub or seal pup but any naturalist can tell you that it is very rare for young to be abandoned by their parents unless the parents have been killed or trapped themselves. If you know for certain that the parents cannot return to their young, even then you should pause before taking action in order to assess the long-term implications of human interference—for yourself as well as for the "orphan". Sometimes, for example, it is best to leave appropriate food for older abandoned cubs at their den or sett, so that they remain in their natural environment and family territory without becoming too trusting of humans, who are so often their enemies.

In late spring and early summer rescue centres sigh in despair at the number of people bringing in little birds with the comment, "I found it in the garden—it couldn't fly—it was all by itself on the lawn." If only they had watched discreetly, they would have seen the parents returning to feed their young once the human "predator" was safely out of the way. Leave fledglings where they are: the parents know all about them. Only interefere if there are cats or other predators around, and then only move the birds carefully into the nearest bush so that they are out of predatory reach but still within their parents' purlieu. Watch for quite a long time to see that the parents have found them. If they have still not been fed after a couple of hours or more, and certainly by nightfall, then and only then should you consider "rescuing" them. There is more about this in Chapter 8.

In the case of young wildlife, you should do a great deal of heart-searching before you become involved in their rescue. Even if you are absolutely certain that the youngster has indeed been deserted for good, stop and think about the next few months ahead. Yes, months—if not years. Hand-rearing a young wild creature is a considerable undertaking, and the younger it is the greater the challenge. You will need abundant time, skill, devotion, patience, consistency and understanding just to feed it and keep it alive, and even then the odds against success are very high indeed. As every farmer knows, even the young of farm animals, accustomed by domestication to close contact with humans, are immediately more prone to disease and disaster when removed from their natural mothers. The mammalian mother passes antibodies to her offspring through her milk; and that milk is of exactly the right composition in terms of fats, protein, vitamins and minerals to be acceptable to the young animal's digestive system and give it maximum benefit. Animal scientists have analysed the milk of farm livestock and of certain zoo species and a limited number of wild native animals so that substitutes can be fed to orphans, but they have not been able to incorporate the vital antibodies that will save the life of a new-born creature, nor to make allowances for the less than perfect hygiene or measuring techniques on many farms. What hope, then, is there for mammalian wildlife? It can be done, but it is never easy.

Can you be sure that there will always be someone on hand to feed the orphan at perhaps two-hourly or even hourly intervals in the early stages? Can you get hold of the right kind of food, be it milk substitutes for mammals, dead day-old chicks for birds of prey and owls, half-digested fish for certain marine birds, or protein-rich insects for other birds?

And then what? If you do succeed in the early stages (which will be something of a miracle in itself), what happens next? The cuddly little cub will grow: it will need meat—more and more meat (preferably regurgitated at first)—and it will need space, and company of its own kind. That pretty little fawn will grow, too, and need a fence at least as tall as a man and a large field, with protection from dogs, and if it is a male it will become dangerous when it matures; the more tame it is, the more likely it is to turn on you (yes, you) in the rutting season, and it could cause severe injury, or even kill a small child.

The helpless little fledgling will soon grow, and stretch its wings and want to fly. It will need to learn how to find its own appropriate food: how do you help, say, a swift or swallow which feeds only as it flies, or how do you teach an owl how to catch a live mouse? And those little rabbits will grow; they will nibble and chew, and will dig, and in an amazingly short time will begin to breed. A female rabbit is sexually mature at only four months old . . .

If you are at all tempted to raise young wildlife yourself, please read Chapter 9 on Rehabilitation before you decide to start. Look to the long term first; that is, once you are absolutely certain that the young animal needs "rescuing" anyway. And then ask for advice and help: telephone an appropriate rescue organisation or centre or a sympathetic veterinary surgeon, explain the circumstances in full detail and listen carefully to the advice. However much personal satisfaction it might give you to hand-rear the creature, put its real needs before your own.

If it is a mistake to act impulsively with wildlife, then the same is equally true when faced with another heart-rending dilemma: the fate of kittens and puppies dumped to die, or sitting forlornly in a pet shop or at a rescue centre. Again, think first. Sweet, cuddly animals grow. Can you continue to care for them when they do so? In the meantime the urge to help and to care will be overwhelming, but you have been warned! Detailed advice on raising orphans of different species can be found in Chapter 8.

Your reactions to injured or trapped creatures (as opposed to orphans) will of course be much more instinctive: you will want to relieve the animal of its distress immediately, and this is one of the principles of first aid. But, once again, think before you act. Assess the situation before you do anything else. It might take less time than a blink for you to decide what to do, but slow down; by charging straight in you could make matters worse for the animal and possibly dangerous for yourself. With wildlife in particular, you should be aware that quite often it is the stress of contact with humans that kills the animal as much as the stress of the original situation. Understanding animal behaviour *before* handling (see Chapter 2) is therefore *as* important, if not more so, than the first-aid procedures themselves, which are described in Chapter 3.

Sometimes it is far kinder to end a suffering animal's life, quickly and humanely, and this very difficult decision is considered in Chapter 5, which also gives guidance on the most humane methods of putting different kinds of animals out of their misery. It is a subject most of us try to avoid but if you take an interest in a distressed creature you must also take responsibility for it and for the quality of the life you want to save.

Quite apart from compassionate and moral consideration in animal rescue, there is also the legal situation. Whilst for the most part the law will not impede emergency rescue, you do need to be fully aware of the implications of the Wildlife and Countryside Act 1981 (known as WCA) in particular, especially if you are handling birds of prey, bats and other protected species. The Act was designed to protect wildlife but sometimes it seems to be unnecessarily obstructive to those whose concern is to rescue and rehabilitate distressed creatures.

A major problem for would-be animal rescuers can be the attitudes of other people, who can in some situations be indignant, abusive or even violent, so that you might need to be not just compassionate for the animal but also understanding, diplomatic, discreet and occasionally invisible. For example, much as you might abhor the use of snares set by gamekeepers, you need to bear in mind that a good keeper will only set snares to catch a specific individual animal—say, a known fox which he believes is raiding the pheasant pens. But however carefully he sites the snare, there is always the risk that other animals will be caught, and those can include badgers, deer, cats and dogs. The keeper might argue that domestic pets should not have been in the area anyway but that is no compensation to the animal. It is a typical human failing to meet criticism (expressed or implied) with a self-defensive hardening of attitude: a confronted keeper might well become more determined to set snares rather than find other ways of protecting the birds on which he has spent so much time and care in rearing.

Even if the whole business of game-rearing is anathema to you, remember that a good keeper can be a great asset to local wildlife. Habitats which suit pheasants suit many other birds and a wide range of mammals as well. Your best hope might be to persuade him that his battle is pointless: any fox he kills will soon be replaced in that territory by another and he might do better to ensure that the pheasant pens are fox-proof and that the birds are encouraged to be self-sufficient before their release, even if that does make them much more wily before the guns. Chicken owners will sympathise with the keeper but, here again, the fault is on the human side rather than the fox's: we create artificial situations, exploiting for our own benefit relatively docile birds which we gather together so that they are unable to escape as they would in the wild. A fox is a natural predator, and no predator could resist such an invitation to dine.

Of course, most gamekeepers set legal snares but it is now illegal to use self-locking snares, or to snare protected species like various raptors, or to use a wide range of other types of trap, whatever the intended victim might be. However, you yourself could be guilty of theft if you remove a snare or trap; the advice of the League Against Cruel Sports, which is totally opposed to the use of any kind of snare, is that if you find one you should either remove it and take it to the nearest police station, or at least render it safe and then report its location to the police *and* the RSPCA so that its legality can be checked. If you hand the snare over to the police, you are unlikely to be charged with theft because there is no apparent intention to "permanently deprive" the owner of the snare.

CONSIDERATION

Cruelty to animals can take many forms, from the deliberate and vicious (badger-digging and dog-fighting), to the unwitting distress which even the most caring of us can inflict without realising. With a little consideration by a lot of people, many animal casualties could be avoided.

Roads

Some accidents are unavoidable unless all traffic moves at a crawl but there are ways of reducing the enormous toll. It might seem obvious that people should drive more carefully on country roads but there is little evidence that they do.

In the case of migratory species, positive action is possible. For example, where adult toads move to their traditional breeding ponds in a great tidal wave lasting several days volunteer naturalists can put themselves on ferry duty for that time, put up "Toads crossing" signs, or make sure that tunnels are built under the road.

Pressure on road-builders at the design stage can also bring benefits for animals such as badgers, whose regular routes can be catered for by building tunnels. Designers also need to cater for deer, and they do so, more for the sake of the motorist than the deer, but still to the benefit of the animal. As signs are generally ignored the only practical method is to erect very high fencing set well back from the road to prevent the deer from straying but, sadly, this cannot be done for every road in the land, even where deer are known to be in residence.

Night is a dangerous time for animals near a road because they are so easily dazzled by headlights, which confuse them or freeze them into immobility in the middle of the road. In addition, moths and other insects are attracted to light, and hunting bats and owls are attracted to the insects: the crunch is inevitable. If you see an animal, wild or domesticated, on or near the road in a country lane, slow right down and at least dip your headlights. It is often necessary to switch them off completely for a minute or two until the animal's eyesight has adjusted.

Railway lines can also be a problem. Where these have been electrified the railway authorities need to be made aware of regular crossing routes, and encouraged to introduce tunnels and bridges or rail-gaps to help the animals across in safety.

Debris and Pollution

It goes without saying that pollutants and poisons cause considerable damage to all creatures, but there is also the problem of our rubbish. For example, birds and small mammals have trouble with aluminium ring-pulls from canned drinks and with plastic collars from can-packs, both of which are snares for the unwary and the innocent, entangling their legs or in some cases lassooing their necks or bodies. Open tins, jars and yogurt pots invite the attentions of a scavenging animal and hedgehogs sometimes quite literally get stuck in—their snouts jammed into the container. Small rodents find their way into unwashed milk bottles and cannot get out again, and old tyres, used to start a fire, leave a lethal tangle of fine wire to entrap an animal. Then, of course, there is all that discarded angling tackle—those fine, almost invisible and quite unbreakable nylon lines that snare little creatures and get swallowed by birds hook, line and sinker, as they say. The situation regarding anglers' weights is slowly improving, though there are still many tons of lead weight lying in the mud or on the banks waiting to be taken as gizzard grit, and out in the woods and fields are many more tons of lead shotgun pellets which can easily be ingested by grazing livestock and birds. And what about those innocent balloons released to celebrate an occasion or to see whose flies furthest? I nearly lost a calf once which, being young and curious, had eaten the remains of a balloon that had drifted unnoticed into its field.

Hot air balloons can also cause terror to creatures on the ground. The combination of a huge, silent shape in the sky like a giant hawk and the sudden whooshing sound as the flame is charged causes livestock to hightail it across the field and deer to bound away in a panic. Dogs and cats have been known to disappear for hours, or to hide trembling in a corner, and there have been cases of sheep and cows aborting their young.

Gardens

Here the hazards are numerous, however innocent their original use or purpose. That fine green nylon netting used to protect fruit crops from birds all too easily entangles them, especially inexperienced fledglings; those strands of black cotton set up to keep birds off seedbeds and flowers can trap birds, small mammals and the occasional unsuspecting toad. Tennis and football nets can catch an unwary hedgehog or badger which has tried to push its way through one of the meshes and got stuck. Then there are poisons like slug pellets (yes, wildlife and pets do sometimes eat them and suffer), rodenticides, insecticides, herbicides, fungicides—stop and think before you spray. The insects are eaten by birds, amphibians and mammals; the leaves are eaten by grazers and browsers. If you use salt on your icy paths, keep it well away from any ponds: it will kill the fish.

Habitat disturbance should also be considered. You might think of it as a compost heap or a potential bonfire, but many other creatures think of it as a warm, safe refuge. Check before you drive your garden fork into a pile of compost or leafmould, and certainly check before you strike a match for a bonfire. Turn over stones with care: there may be a toad underneath and in spring, take care with your mowing—you are liable to mince up thumbnail-sized toadlets and froglets which thought they were safe in the jungle.

Another garden hazard is the pond, or a swimming pool. Both can have steep sides making it quite impossible for an animal that has fallen in to get out again, so make sure that ponds have at least one gently sloping bank. Empty pools and ponds can also be a hazard to a small animal like a hedgehog which falls in and cannot climb out again, so make sure there is an escape ramp.

Farms

On the farm, water tanks can be fatally attractive to owls, but a piece of wood floating on the water will enable them to extricate themselves. Cattle-grids are very often traps for hedgehogs and should always incorporate an escape ramp. Baler twine is a double risk as it can either ensnare or be eaten by livestock.

Hay-making and harvesting are highly dangerous times for all manner of wildlife, especially ground-nesting birds (pheasants, larks etc. and the young of lying-up species like deer and hares, let alone the countless small mammals that have been living undisturbed among the corn crops. Hedge-trimming is another farm activity which needs to be carried out with consideration and careful timing in order to cause the minimum of disruption to sheltering, berry-eating or nesting birds. Hedge removal can be the naturalist's nightmare: hedgerows are essential highways for wildlife, enabling birds and mammals to move safely between habitats and also supplying a considerable larder of food for many species. Farmers who are concerned for wildlife can get plenty of helpful and practical advice from their county FWAG (Farming and Wildlife Advisory Groups) advisor who is likely to have a background in agriculture as well as conservation and will understand the problems.

And then there is one of the major hazards to be found on farms and in many gardens: the domestic cat. Unfortunately, whether the cat is a fireside pet or a barn ratter, it is an unparalleled killer and injurer of wildlife. Nearly every wildlife rescue centre in the country finds that the great majority of its casualties have had an argument either with a car or with a cat.

Habitat

An animal cannot survive without a suitable habitat, and where humans have not literally destroyed habitats they have created hazards within them. For example, power lines stretching across open countryside are a frequent death trap for large, cumbersome fliers like swans, or uncertain and ungainly young herons, and even an agile hawk can collide with a familiar cable when it is intent on its prey.

The luckier birds are killed outright; the unfortunate lose a leg, or a wing, or are crippled by the impact and crash to the ground to die slowly or to be taken by a scavenging predator. The problem is of particular significance for swans and the Swan Rescue Service in Norfolk has been trying to persuade electricity boards to avoid putting any more electricity pylons across known swan flight paths, and preferably to bury cables rather than string them up in the air, or at the very least festoon them with warning discs that would be more visible in foggy conditions.

The essential activities of foresters can be enormously destructive of habitats, but many of them are conservationists and naturalists and will do all in their power to minimise the harmful effects of forestry, including keeping an eye out for nesting birds and bats roosting in hollow trees. Owls often use tree hollows too and all these species can be helped by leaving old trees standing and then making sure that the hollows are not waterlogged. If there are not enough natural holes around, a carefully planned installation of appropriate nesting and roosting boxes for birds and bats is invaluable.

Gardens are increasingly a refuge for wildlife, and all the more so if some part of the garden is left rough and undisturbed. A large proportion of our amphibians now rely on garden ponds, and very many birds rely heavily on gardens for shelter and food. The winter bird table must have had a considerable effect on the number of birds which survive the season, and it is thought that something like two-thirds of our blue tit population owes its survival to peanuts! Cater for some of the larger birds too by putting out meaty bones, chicken carcases etc. for corvids and other meat-eaters. However, winter feeding can also cause disease, injury and death: avoid the slightest hint of mould on food (especially peanuts), and place the feeding point well out of reach of lurking cats. Many small birds are at the mercy of sparrowhawks, too, although the sparrowhawk kills only to survive and deserves a winter dining table as much as any other bird.

Pets

It is hardly necessary to advise the kind of person who reads this book on how to care for a domestic pet, but there are several points which need to be stressed. The first, and most obvious, is: never buy or adopt a pet on impulse. Secondly, responsible pet owners should habitually have their domestic animals neutered unless they are specifically to be used for selective breeding. Such action would take a considerable load off the welfare centres and would substantially reduce the worrying increase in stray and feral cats and dogs.

Not all strays are unwanted offspring: many dogs are "latchkey" pets allowed to roam freely by irresponsible owners. Even if they have been neutered so that there is no risk of unwanted puppies, if allowed to roam freely they are still capable of causing road accidents, upsetting dustbins, depositing faeces on the pavement, urinating in children's playgrounds, chasing cats, biting children, attacking other dogs, frightening horse-riders and worrying livestock. If you have ever seen the results of a dog's raid on a meek flock of sheep or precious angora goats, you will understand the rage and revulsion that causes even the most dog-loving shepherd to get out a gun and shoot the dog on the spot (and quite legally). Perhaps people do not realise that *any* dog is capable of worrying sheep, however docile it may be at home or however well trained it is in your company. There can only be one solution to this problem if you want to show your compassion for animals: start by taking responsibility for your own pets.

CHAPTER TWO

ANIMAL BEHAVIOUR AND HANDLING TECHNIQUES

EMERGENCY CHECKLIST

- Be calmly efficient, and firm but gentle.

- Keep all your movements smooth and sure.

- Keep your eyes averted: a direct gaze is threatening.

- Keep other people well away unless their help is essential.

- Protect yourself: wear gloves; beware of horns, hooves, teeth, claws, talons; keep your face out of reach.

- Most creatures are quieter in darkness: hoods, blindfolds and dark containers are invaluable aids.

- Use only as much restraint as is necessary to protect the animal or the handler, or to transport the animal if that is essential. Try the kindest methods first.

- Guide or lure rather than chase an animal into confinement.

- Be prepared: keep basic equipment handy (especially in the car) and use your imagination to improvise.

- IF YOU DO NOT FEEL CONFIDENT IN HANDLING A SITUATION, GET HELP FROM SOMEONE WHO CAN COPE.

All animals, whether wild or domesticated, retain at least a vestige of suspicion of human beings, particularly of those they do not know. Man represents a threat—sometimes specifically because of his species but at other times simply by being a stranger—and the natural reaction of any animal is either to hide or to flee. If both prove impossible, then fear will prompt the animal to fight in self-defence, and a frightened animal can be far more vicious than an aggressive one. It is vital, therefore, that your initial approach and subsequent handling of an animal are made in full awareness of its fear of the situation.

Those with experience of domesticated livestock know that the most successful approach to most animals is to be calm and firm but gentle. Some, such as bulls, do need more dominant handling but most farm animals, accustomed to some degree of proximity with humans, generally respond better to quiet self-confidence than to aggressive dominance or apprehension. This is true in familiar situations, and the more so if the animal is in distress.

Wild animals, including those which are born in captivity or are accustomed to enclosure, are always placed under considerable stress by the unfamiliarity of humans at close quarters (or perhaps an unfortunate familiarity through traumatic encounters in the past) and if the animal is also either trapped, sick or hurt the stress caused by a human presence is multiplied alarmingly. In some cases your presence alone is enough to cause fatal shock—and that is before you have made any positive moves at all.

Stress has been defined by its acronym: Situations That Release Emergency Signals for Survival. To that end, stress is essential to any living creature if it wishes to remain alive, but when stress becomes damaging it becomes distress. If an animal's instinct to hide or flee from a situation it distrusts, especially if a human is involved, is thwarted by circumstance, then it is immediately in a state of distress.

It is sad but true that most animals consider humans to be predatory enemies, and there is no reason for an animal to assume that you are any different to any other human predator. Your first task, therefore, is to offer reassurance that your intentions are benevolent. Very few people have the absolute empathy with animals that allows them to instil confidence by their own body language and if you are one of those people you do not need any books to guide you. You will know instinctively what to do.

Every animal, human or otherwise, has an invisible capsule of space around it within which it feels safe. If this "flight distance" is invaded, it reacts by either literally or metaphorically escaping, or, if escape is not possible, by fighting. Social species adjust to the close presence of other, familiar members of their own species but still maintain their flight distance in the case of strangers of their own species or potential predators of any species, including man. "Flight" includes running or flying away, hiding in a burrow or withdrawing into the safety of a shell or a spiny coat. It also includes the strange phenomenon of "freezing", whereby the animal hopes to escape the notice of a predator or opponent, or, if already capured, might fall into the profound state of unresponsiveness which is termed "tonic immobility" and is very like a hypnotic trance, in which the animal is aware of what is going on but seems to be incapable of responding. This trance-like state is seen in every kind of animal from insects to mammals and birds, as though instinct tells them there is at least a possibility that, as most predators lose interest in motionless prey, the victim might be released and escape its fate. The possum playing dead just has to hope that the hunter does not intend to eat its prey as soon as it is "dead", and indeed it is not unusual for a death-feigning duck to be buried by a fox for later consumption and be able to make a successful escape from its grave. Watch out, too, for the animal which seems to accept you passively and willingly: its panic will be revealed by its eyes, those barometers of stress, which might have a wild look to them, or be moving with excessive rapidity or, on the contrary, staring fixedly or dull and glazed.

If escape, whether by fleeing, hiding or bluffing, is impossible or fails, the animal's last resort is retaliation against the predator, perhaps by hissing and spitting, by ejecting some foul substance or smell, or by fighting back with whatever weapons are available—teeth, claws, talons, beak, horns and so on. The will to live lends considerable strength and courage to this defensive attack, whatever the odds. Bearing in mind that you, intending to be the saviour of a distressed animal, are more than likely to be regarded as a predator, you should be aware that these retaliatory fear-driven attacks can be very vicious and in some cases can cause you considerable damage. For example, a bird of prey might seem to be incapacitated and although you have wisely taken precautions to prevent it from attacking you with its fearsome beak it will still take you by surprise by lying on its back and slashing with powerful, sharp talons that can rip ribbons of flesh from your hands. Even a hare or rabbit can damage you with a few strong kicks from its back feet, raking you with its claws. A roe buck might use its horns like other deer but the doe will surprise you by "boxing" with her front feet, and her cleats, as sharp as flint tools and driven at you with powerful kicks, are even more effective than the raptor's slash. Several horned species box and kick if cornered, finding their hooves more effective than horns.

Never, ever, put your face near any distressed animal, however small, feeble or incapacitated it seems to be: you might easily end up blind. Remember that a wild animal has no reason at all to trust any human being; it will assume your intentions are to take advantage of its situation, and even the most loving domesticated dog or cat might attack its owner if it has been badly injured and shocked in a road accident and feels vulnerable. Domesticated animals are not so different from their wild ancestors when they feel at risk. The same applies with many maternal creatures: the tamest bitch can be as aggressively protective of her litter as the wildest wolf.

Always remember that, first and foremost, you are seen as a predator. In most cases, prey species have their eyes at the sides of their heads for a wider angle of vision to detect the approach of predator species, which usually have forward-facing eyes, like our own. If a stuffed hawk is presented to chickens, the birds react as if it is a live hawk, but if the stuffed bird's eyes are covered, they will ignore it. And if a pair of hawk-like eyes are presented to them without any body at all, they still react as if it is a live hawk.

Eyes play an important role in body language and you should avoid looking an animal direct in the eye or staring steadily in its direction. Indeed, keep your eyes averted whenever you can. In the case of canids, for example, bold eye contact is usually taken as aggression or dominance: think how "embarrassed" a dog (or cat) becomes under a steady look. For prey animals, eyes are particularly alarming. Think of the sheepdog fixing a flock with its eye in the same way as the ancestral wolf immobilises a wild herd; think of the steady, piercing stare of an unblinking raptor or a hunting cat. All animals recognise a human partly by the round face, as well as the upright stance, and in order to approach a wild animal you need to reduce your stance and camouflage your give-away face by breaking up its outline or making use of a hat pulled well down.

Many animals seem to assume that if you are not looking straight at them you are unaware of them and they are safe. A fox, intent on other business, can pass close to pheasants without disturbing them in the least: they seem to appreciate that it is not their turn to be the prey. A person can walk into a field of grazing rabbits with eyes averted and often be able to stroll almost within arm's reach of them. A hare will sit and watch you in some bemusement if you steadily walk around it in decreasing circles, and in theory you can so mesmerise it that you can simply pick it up when you reach the centre of your spiral. However, it is highly unlikely that you will actually catch rabbits and hares in these situations! The oblique approach can be interpreted as a sneaky attack as much as an aimless meander, and the animals are very much on their guard.

Another typical reaction of an animal is that if it cannot see you it feels safe: your presence is almost forgotten. Many species are immediately quietened by being plunged suddenly into darkness and one of the more useful items of equipment in rescue work is your own clothing. Drop a shirt or light sweater over a small animal, or a jacket over the head of a larger one, and it will stay still and be much easier to handle. This technique applies to, for example, large animals like cattle, horses and deer (which can all be blindfolded to calm them down), cats, and even badgers (for a short while, if you are lucky). It also works with most birds, though you need to adjust the size of the "blanket" to suit the size of the bird. Use a handkerchief for a small passerine, for example, or a piece of dark cloth for a corvid, or a black bag-net for a pheasant or chicken, which will produce an instant black-out and not only traps the bird but stops it even wanting to move. The quickest way of calming a henhouse full of agitated biddies is to turn out the lights.

Light can also be used positively in some circumstances. A nocturnal or crepuscular creature is all too easily blinded by sudden artificial lighting (hence so many road casualties) and you can sometimes use a strong torch to transfix a deer, a rabbit or an owl in order to catch it.

Preliminaries to the act of capture often make a bad situation worse, especially if the victim is at all mobile. Instead of chasing, which is a predatory act, try to shepherd the animal steadily and quietly into a position where it can be more readily caught. That is not at all easy in wide open spaces, especially if you are alone and the creature is well aware of your intentions. Use your ingenuity, which is the most useful tool and art an animal rescuer can possess. In some cases, however, it is important to make the capture in the shortest possible time to avoid undue stress and this might be better achieved if there are several people involved, particularly in the case of, say, oiled birds whose one intention is to return to the water.

With a creature already in distress, shepherding must be very gentle and subtle but not hesitant. In a garden, it should be relatively easy to corner the animal by a wall or fence, or to edge it very gradually into a shed. But take care: an animal might well try to go to ground *under* a shed instead and will be difficult to dislodge.

However familiar you might be with a particular species, every animal is an individual and every situation is unique. I can only give the broadest of guidelines on handling animals; your own experience and intuition will help you choose the best course of action in each case. In any situation in which you do not feel confident about handling a distressed animal, call someone who does rather than making the situation worse for the animal. Later in this chapter there are sections devoted to the handling of different species, but first of all here are some of the basics of handling any animal, wild or domesticated, in any situation.

If you come across a wild animal in unusual circumstances—out in the open in broad daylight, for example, or in a position from which it cannot easily escape—do not just bless your luck at the privilege of seeing it at all but be very suspicious. Keep well back and motionless while you assess the situation. Bearing in mind that a distressed animal's reaction to your approach might be to freeze, escape or fight, and that you are more than likely to be recognised as a potential predator, your aim must be to cause the least distress. Aim for minimal handling in the shortest possible time but ensure that your handling is positive, steady and kind. It nearly always helps if you talk quietly to an animal, keeping up a low conversation which most creatures, wild or tame, will find reassuring to some degree. Keep all your movements smooth and deliberate, with no sudden or hesitant gestures and no loud noises, hisses or rustling of waterproof clothing.

Take a couple of deep breaths to steady your own nerves, because if you are at all nervous you will only heighten the animal's anxiety. Try to be predictable: remember that predators are unpredictable, making sudden attacking movements. This is particularly important with domesticated animals, who are always happiest in known routines and circumstances.

Above all, perhaps, be firm but gentle. Those who handle horses are well aware of the importance of "gentling" a nervous animal with a soothing voice and assured stroking. Horses, hens and dogs, for example, can be stroked almost into a trance, and a tame ferret can be transformed from a struggling bundle of energy wanting to be somewhere else into an elongated and totally relaxed dangle of fur if you hold it under the elbows and quietly and repetitively stroke its knuckles. It will be asleep in no time.

RESTRAINT

It is important to be able to restrain a casualty, partly so that it does not attack you but mainly to protect it from causing itself more damage. Restraint should be limited: use only as much as is necessary to prevent further self-injury, to give first aid without injury to the handler, and to transport the animal to the veterinary surgery or place of safety. Consider restraint, which includes catching, as the essential initial step in first aid.

Wherever possible, try luring or shepherding rather than chasing an animal; better still, provide a situation into which it will retire of its own accord. For shepherding, it is usually best to work on the funnelling principle, gradually guiding the animal into an increasingly restricted space so that it ends up where you want it, almost without realising it. If you are confining larger wild mammals in a garden shed for want of anywhere else in an emergency, take special care to black out the windows and ensure they cannot be smashed. If you are using a loose-box, bear in mind that a wild animal will probably do its best to get out by clambering, smashing or digging, and the same applies to pens and other enclosures. Ensure that the animal has privacy and that part of the holding area allows it to disappear from sight so that it feels more secure.

Watch out for sick or frightened animals of some species going to ground under a shed—they might die if left lying up. Sometimes a shepherd's crook can encourage them out, or in extreme cases it might be necessary to remove a few floorboards, working quietly so that the animal is not alarmed. Be prepared for it to bolt.

Make full use of certain animals' desire to go to ground: it is often quite easy to lure them into a dark, enclosed space like a stout carrying box. Once they are in, they will relax, especially if they believe their confinement is voluntary.

Other animals, especially herbivores, are wary of enclosed structures and would much prefer to be out in the open, albeit shielded by shrubbery or the contours of the land. Cattle, for example, spook readily at shadowy places; sheep instinctively head up a slope rather than down, and towards daylight rather than into darkness; horses might refuse to enter an open-fronted field shelter voluntarily even in the foulest weather. It is often easier to lead than drive such animals: they sometimes follow you out of curiosity more readily than be herded ahead of you, especially if you have some food rattling in a tin bowl. With luck, even deer can be attracted in this way. However, sick animals of any species are unlikely to be in the least interested in food lures.

In most cases you will need to confine the animal to some extent for treatment, recuperation and observation, or to transport it for further treatment after first aid. The essence of any container for these purposes is that it should confine the animal in such a way that its injuries are not aggravated, it is calmed and reassured, it can be safely transported, and it cannot injure its handler.

The simplest container is a coat, jacket or sweater wrapped over and around the animal. A garment can be used to restrict limb movements of smaller animals and to give the darkness that quietens so many of them. It also provides warmth in the initial treatment of shock, and deflects attempted bites and scratches. And it is likely to be the only equipment to hand in an emergency.

A hessian sack is even better. Many animals can be popped into a sack where they will be warm and in the dark and will be less likely to cause themselves further damage. Even a badger will go quiet—for a short while—if a thick sack is dropped over it. Large birds often travel well in sacks, too, and can have their heads and necks protruding while the rest of the body is confined within.

Cardboard boxes are ideal for transporting and accommodating smaller creatures like cats, and are excellent for most birds, which are much happier than in a cage because they feel securely invisible and are not alarmed by being able to see sudden movements outside their sanctuary. Boxes are also warmer and draught-free, and provide subdued light and privacy.

For the animal's own sense of security, it does help to use a container that can subsequently become part of its emergency accommodation while it is recuperating. This is especially true for wild animals, who will be bewildered by the new environment and territory. The container in which they have travelled to that environment will have become familiar during the journey and is a substitute for the burrow, den, earth or roost they have been forced to leave.

To sum up: only restrain to the degree necessary and always try the kindest methods first by reassurance and firm but gentle handling. Choose the safe minimum so that the victim is not subjected to any greater stress than necessary, because all too often it is the stress of handling, not the original injury or situation, that kills or prolongs recovery.

In emergencies, act quickly, be efficient and firm, but above all be calm, kind and predictable. If other people are present, especially the owner of an injured domestic animal, they too will benefit from your cool and competent attitude—and people often need as much reassurance as the animal casualty. In most circumstances you should keep other people well out of the way and out of the animal's sight and hearing, except where another pair of hands is essential.

EQUIPMENT

Well-armed animals need very careful handling, for your sake as much as theirs, and you would be well advised to find or devise some appropriate equipment. At the very least, even if you never expect to find an animal casualty of any kind, it would help to have some basic items in your vehicle at all times—especially a pair of thick leather gloves, some form of "blanket" (old jacket, sheet etc.), a makeshift "rope", a sharp knife and a pair of wire-cutters, and a container such as a strong cardboard box or even a zip-up hold-all.

Ropes

It is often necessary to bind or hobble the legs of an animal, either to prevent its escape or to prevent it from lashing out and breaking its own limbs or injuring a handler. To hobble a large herbivore like a horse, cow or deer, link two legs by tying a rope just above the fetlocks. Ideally you need something strong but soft to avoid chafing and bruising—likely emergency "ropes" include neckties, knotted handkerchiefs, nylon tights, bandages, a dog's leash, leather belts and woollen scarves. Baler twine is strong but is liable to cut into the animal's flesh. Out in the wilds with absolutely nothing

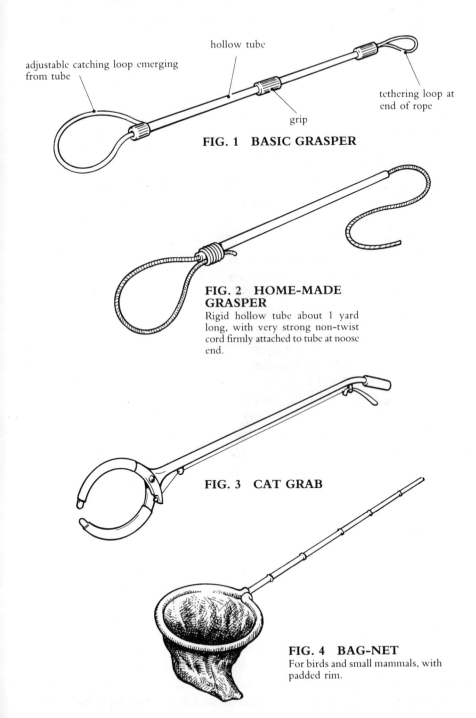

hollow tube

adjustable catching loop emerging
from tube

tethering loop at
end of rope

grip

FIG. 1   BASIC GRASPER

**FIG. 2   HOME-MADE
GRASPER**
Rigid hollow tube about 1 yard
long, with very strong non-twist
cord firmly attached to tube at noose
end.

FIG. 3   CAT GRAB

FIG. 4   BAG-NET
For birds and small mammals, with
padded rim.

in your pockets and not even a pair of socks to use, try twisting and plaiting long grasses, reeds or rushes. Ivy or woodbine vines would need padding.

Grasper

To catch and restrain an aggressive animal (for example, a dog, cat, fox, otter, badger) speed will probably be critical: you need a quick, clean catch in the interests of efficiency and the elimination of stress. Try a grasper, either bought or home-made, and practise with it on a fence post so that you feel confident in its use during an emergency. You can buy a variety of graspers—the Dutch make the UNO Ketch-All pole, for example, in a range of sizes, and some British companies make or distribute animal graspers designed for cats and dogs (see Fig. 1). To make your own, you need a hollow metal rod strong enough not to bend in use: try a 3-foot length of copper pipe about an inch or an inch-and-a-quarter in diameter. Take about 8 feet of plastic-covered cable, fold it in half and slip the folded end through the tube so that it protrudes as a loop at the other end. Tie the loose ends in a knot to prevent the cable being pulled right through the tube when the animal is caught (see Fig. 2). As a refinement, use a piece of steel tube ending in a Y-joint at the loop end; then the metal Y helps to control the animal as well.

Slip the adjustable loop over the animal's head and round its neck without throttling it (catch a forelimb as well if you can), then use the rigidity of the pole to keep the animal at arm's length or to persuade it into a prone position if it is really dangerous. The loop can be slackened from the safe distance of the other end of the pole. It is essential that the pole is strong enough not to bend or break when you are handling an active and determined animal, and some of the manufactured cat- and dog-graspers will not be able to deal with an angry badger.

The grasper can also be used to lift a spitting ball-of-fury cat at arm's length and drop it carefully into a container for closer restraint or transport. An alternative for cats is a pair of tongs, or cat-grab (see Fig. 3). For much smaller creatures—certain rodents, reptiles and invertebrates—use long forceps with padded rubber tips.

Do not use a grasper on a timid animal of any species unless you really have no other option: it will find the equipment frightening.

Muzzle

You will almost certainly need to muzzle a wild carnivore for your own protection, if you can get near enough to do so. To restrain a long-muzzled animal (for example, most dogs, foxes and otters, but not cats or badgers) and prevent it from biting, use a length of suitable material (rope, leather leash or belt, necktie, bandage, scarf, nylon tights) about 3 feet long. Form a loose loop; slip it over the animal's jaws with the knot on top of the muzzle. Tighten it gently but firmly to bind the jaws, cross the loose ends under the throat and then tie them at the back of the animal's head behind the ears (see Fig. 5). Do not use a muzzle if the jaw has been injured.

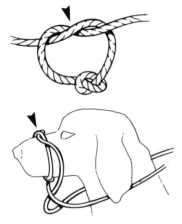

FIG. 5   MUZZLING A DOG
1. Make a loop loose enough to go over dog's muzzle. If using makeshift "rope", tie an under-chin knot.
2. Slip loop over muzzle, with free ends on top.
3. Take free ends down either side, cross under lower jaw, then tie firmly at back of head.

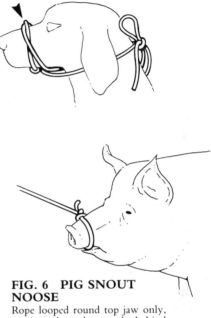

FIG. 6   PIG SNOUT NOOSE
Rope looped round top jaw only, passing through mouth behind tusks.

Checks

A check is simply a chain or leash which works something like a free-running snare: if the animal struggles, the noose tightens around the neck, but relaxes when the animal stops resisting. A check chain (sometimes unfortunately called a choke chain) is a length of chain with a ring at one end through which the other end is passed to form a loop. The ring should be such that the chain slides easily through it. An ordinary leather or nylon dog leash can be used instead: slip the free (clip) end of the leash through its handle-loop to make the noose.

Crook

The traditional shepherd's crook is now made in aluminium alloy for lightness, strength and flexibility and can be obtained from good farm suppliers. Ideally about 4 feet long, it is also called a leg catcher or swan hook and is an all-purpose tool. It can be used to hook a hiding animal out of an awkward place, or to capture sheep, goats and pigs by the leg, or large birds like swans and geese by the neck. Do not use on deer: their legs are much too vulnerable. Also beware of bruising on sheep's legs and with lambs use the crook at the neck.

To catch a swan or goose, hook the crook around the bird's neck and twist the crook a little to prevent the bird slipping its head free. Then draw the bird towards you firmly until you can take hold of it manually.

Traps

To catch an elusive or difficult animal without injuring it, it is often better to tempt or shepherd it into a confined space rather than try and catch it with a grasper, lariat or tongs. Occasionally it might be appropriate to resort to a "live" or humane trap, that is, one that catches an animal for subsequent release unharmed. Beware of traps with wire mesh sides: many animals lacerate their muzzles, break their teeth or wrench their claws in a desperate attempt to escape.

Longworth Trap (mice, voles, shrews) This is the most widely used trap for the field study of small mammals. Made of aluminium, it has a tunnel leading through a trip-door to a large nest box where the animal can be given bedding and food (see Fig. 7). Similar American traps are the Sherman (sheet aluminium) and the Havahart (wire mesh). There is also the much cheaper, simpler plastic version for indoor use, called the Trip Trap (see Fig. 8), but this must be emptied soon after the creature is caught as it does not have much room for food and bedding.

Live box and cage traps (weasel, stoat, mink, ferret, rabbit, grey squirrel, rat, fox, coypu, feral cat etc.) These also operate on the principle of a trip-door—either a guillotine drop-door or a spring-loaded one, triggered by a treadle or trip-wire, or a one-way "cat-flap" swing door. The Forestry Commission can give details of numerous designs for squirrel traps.

Live bird traps There is a range of cage and pen traps for birds, especially corvids, pigeons and pheasants. The bird enters through a mesh funnel or "letter-box" flap or a treadle-triggered drop-door.

Halters

A simple rope halter has a small knot loop at one end, through which the other end of the rope is passed to form a noose (see Fig. 10). The noose is placed loosely around the animal's neck, with the knot under its chin. Draw the noose tighter, with its top just behind the animal's ears, then pass the loose end of the rope from the small loop over the animal's muzzle and under the noose rope on the left side of the animal's face. If such a halter is used to tie an animal to a solid object, you must use a quick-release knot in case the animal falls. Even so the halter is pretty uncomfortable: when the animal pulls away from the restraint, the rope tends to tighten quite painfully around its muzzle and puts pressure against the back of its ears. It is better to use a proper halter, which might be of rope, leather or flat nylon like a dog's lead. If you are trying to hold a nervous animal on the end of a rope attached to any kind of halter, do *not* wrap the loose end round your hand but pass it behind your back to take the strain. Ropes can burn your hand unpleasantly. (See Figs 11, 12 and 13 for makeshift halters for bulls, calves and horses.)

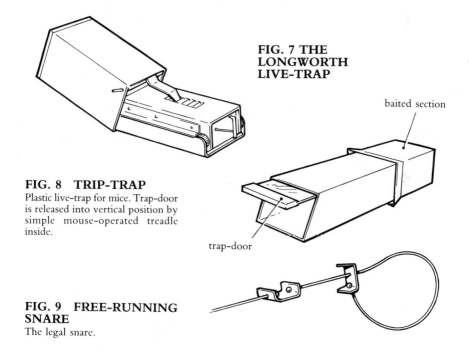

FIG. 7 THE LONGWORTH LIVE-TRAP

baited section

FIG. 8   TRIP-TRAP
Plastic live-trap for mice. Trap-door is released into vertical position by simple mouse-operated treadle inside.

trap-door

FIG. 9   FREE-RUNNING SNARE
The legal snare.

Bag-nets

A bag-net is simply a piece of material, preferably black for instant darkness, attached to a wire loop to form a bag in the shape of a child's shrimping net but large enough to catch up a bird (see Fig. 4). The loop is secured to a handle, usually bamboo for lightness and flexibility.

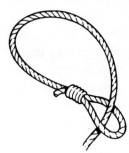

FIG. 10   MAKING A HALTER
Make a small secure noose, then a large loop.

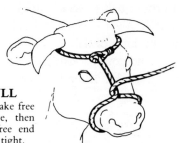

FIG. 11   FOR A BULL
Slip loop around horns. Take free end down centre of face, then around jaws; then slip free end under face rope and draw tight.

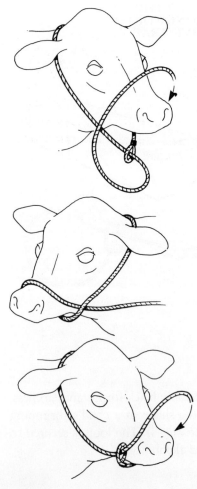

FIG. 12   FOR A CALF
Slip large loop loosely around calf's neck, with noose under throat. Take up slack and, with noose against one side of jaw, take free end over and run it under loop on other side. Draw tight enough to secure.

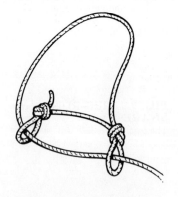

FIG. 13   FOR A HORSE
Make two nooses, one near rope end and the other 4 in from it. Run free end through both nooses. The 4 in section goes over horse's muzzle; first part of large loop behind ears; and last part (running through the nooses) under chin.

Landing-nets

Typical angler's landing-nets can be used to catch all manner of birds and small animals by dropping the net over the creature. One problem is entanglement: do beware of making the animal panic and getting itself inextricably tied up with the netting.

Gloves

Gloves are essential for handling many animals. With biters and scratchers you need a really thick, strong pair of gloves and even then there is a risk of teeth or talons penetrating to your hand—but at least the blows will be deflected and with luck you will only be bruised rather than have your skin lacerated or punctured. Make sure you have kept up your anti-tetanus jabs.

Throw-overs and Blindfolds

Many creatures can be both restrained and calmed if they are placed under cover. Use whatever you have: your jacket, sweater, shirt or other clothing, or a handkerchief or piece of cloth for a small bird, or a hessian sack—anything that will cover a small creature or at least cover the head (especially eyes) of a larger one. As soon as the animal is under cover (so that it cannot see you and believes you cannot see it) and preferably in darkness or very subdued light, it will quieten down. Many animals can then be gathered up with the throw-over still enveloping them, and carried in it in a vehicle or transferred to some other container for transport and treatment.

Blanket Stretcher

A blanket or ground sheet is a useful part of the rescuer's equipment. Quite apart from replacing a jacket as a cover-up for larger animals, it can also be used to move an injured animal up to the size of, say, a roe deer. Once you are certain that careful removal is advisable (see Chapter 3 on First Aid), lay the blanket beside the casualty and very gently lift the bulk of the body on to it, supporting the animal's head and rear quarters. In most cases two people can easily carry such a stretcher.

HANDLING MAMMALS

Badgers

Badgers are shy, deliberate, slow-moving animals. They are also courageous and powerful, and can be dangerous if provoked though they would prefer to run away rather than fight. Because of their strength and tenacity, you should not attempt to handle any badger, however distressed, unless you have experience or are desperate. Otherwise seek professional assistance: a tranquillising dart will make the situation much easier for all concerned, including the badger.

Badgers' teeth are very sharp, enough to snap off your finger, and their strong jaws are self-locking: it is almost impossible to prise them apart once they have taken a hold. No glove is tough enough to withstand the bite of a badger, and you should also keep your ankles well out of the way of its teeth. Its claws, though not used aggressively, are long and sharp enough to do you considerable damage if you happen to be in their way.

Treat any badger with considerable respect. If you find an injured one, it is probably some distance from home: its instinct would be to crawl back to its sett and lie up, either to wait until its wounds heal or to die. If you find it out in the open, it is too badly hurt to retire to its sett.

However, if it is a road casualty it might only be stunned and therefore unconscious. If you can see no superficial injuries and have no reason to suspect internal ones or fractures, the wisest course might be to ease it on to an old jacket and drag it off the highway into the nearest field—preferably on the same side of the road as a known sett. Put it at the base of a hedge, cover it with camouflage vegetation and leave it to come round. Then it will be in familiar territory. Once you remove a badger from its territory, you are immediately faced with considerable problems in rehabilitation (see Chapter 9).

If there is any possibility of internal injury or if there is obvious evidence of external ones or of fractures, you need to bring a veterinary surgeon to the badger. These animals do have remarkable powers of recovery: the Gwent Badger Group claims that badgers allowed to go to ground in their own setts with really quite severe injuries can go into something of a coma for a week or two while the wounds heal themselves. But is that a risk you can let the animal take? If it does try and escape to reach its sett, it would perhaps be better to corner it wherever you can, preferably in a shed or garage, and once it is in there, shut the door: on no account enter the building with it but get expert help.

On the other hand, badgers greatly resent being handled or confined. When you approach an injured badger, it will probably crouch with its nose to the ground in apparent submission, hoping you will go away again. But the moment you touch it—watch out! Unless you are certain that it is unconscious, it is essential to keep your distance and it is preferable to persuade it into a darkened container rather than to try and restrain it with graspers or anything else. If you can offer it a dark bolt-hole like a large box, tea-chest or dustbin on its side with the opening mostly covered with a cloth, it will probably dash in gratefully. If it is caught in a snare, very carefully back it into a container before you make any attempt to remove the wire. Once it is in a dark hiding place, it will be quiet. If nothing else is handy, try dropping a hessian sack or coat over a trapped badger: with luck it will be quiet for just long enough for you to remove the trap.

A badger shut in a shed will probably make frantic efforts to escape and you must get veterinary help as quickly as possible. If you have to transport the animal to the surgery, make sure the container has solid sides (with airholes) so that the badger remains hidden in the dark, and also that it is strong enough to contain the animal if it panics. Telephone the vet in advance to give warning of what is on its way: it will be almost impossible to treat a badger at all, even for superficial problems, without a general anaesthetic or at least very heavy sedation.

There *are* ways of handling a badger but only if it is absolutely essential to do so. You can use a strong grasper with a Y-joint at its noose end, or you might be able to use a very strong net on a tubular frame. A snared badger can be held down by a strong person with the aid of a pitchfork—put a prong on either side of the animal's body (from behind so you are well away from its bite) and anchor it there if you can, much in the same way that a snake might be held down with a forked stick. This method is suggested by the National Animal Rescue Association (NARA) in its excellent first-aid guide, but with the warning that it will take much more strength than you might think. If the snare is around its neck, it could become unconscious and might even need artificial respiration in extreme cases, though sometimes all that is needed is a few minutes of peace and quiet in a box once you have removed the wire. Another trick when dealing with a snared badger is to distract it by giving it a stout stick to clamp its jaws on instead of your arm. Then drop a jacket over its head before you get to work on its release.

Many mammals can be grabbed by the loose skin on the scruff of the neck but do not try that with a badger—there is no neck scruff. However, there is loose skin on the back towards the rump if you need an extra hold.

Bats

All species of bat are carefully protected by the Wildlife and Countryside Act 1981. In theory, you should never touch a bat unless you are licensed to do so: you should call in a member of your local bat group, whose telephone number is available from the Nature Conservancy Council (NCC). In practice, you can legally tend a disabled bat in order to release it as soon as it has recovered, and you can remove a bat to a place of safety if it is in imminent danger from predators.

To pick up any bat, slip your hand under its body and be careful not to hold its wings, which are quite easily damaged. When you offer it a vertical surface, it is more than likely to turn itself upside down and hang head downwards in typical bat fashion, gripping the surface with its hind feet.

Bats become torpid during the day—do not assume that a bat is sick or even dead because it does not seem to react to you. A bat's body temperature drops from 42 °C in flight to somewhere around the ambient temperature of its environment when it is at rest and, like a bumblebee, it needs to warm up by shivering before it can fly again. This could take half an hour or so. A grounded bat might find it very difficult to take off, even when it has warmed up, so lift it up to a branch.

Bats can bite defensively on being handled and it is therefore advisable to wear soft leather gloves if you are unsure of them, or you can put a cloth over the bat and gather it up in a loose bag. On the other hand, many bats do not object to handling at all and soon become very amenable, enjoying a gentle stroke, and they are quite happy to lie in the palm of your hand, or perhaps hang upside down from your finger. If they need to be transported, put them in a *dark* box and have a cling-perch inside it so that they can travel comfortably in true bat style.

Only take in a bat if absolutely necessary: please read Chapter 9 on Rehabilitation to understand the potential problems. The most common injuries are cat-inflicted damage to the wing membranes; a hole will heal itself in due course, but a tear on the edge will be very difficult to make good.

Cats

A distressed cat can lash out with teeth and claws and can cause its handler quite severe damage, the lacerations often becoming infected. Even the friendliest domestic cat can react savagely if it is in pain or frightened, and it will be very difficult to restrain. It is an athletic, supple animal and good at twisting itself out of your grasp.

If you have a cat of your own, get it used to being handled in the security of the home in case it ever needs veterinary treatment. Kneel on an unslippery floor behind the cat, wedging its body between your thighs. Take hold of its neck scruff and press downwards so that its head is safely immobilised, with your forearms bearing down on its back for further control.

A distressed cat is a different matter. *Always* wear gloves to handle a cat in trouble, and get the animal into close confinement immediately: wrap it in a jacket, put it in a hessian sack or in a lidded box with air-holes, or a cage, a cat-basket or even a zip-up hold-all with ventilation. Veterinary surgeons have special cat-carrying cartons which are invaluable; pet shops offer cat-baskets and cat-cages. Watch out for cat claws striking through a cage's sides, though, and make sure that the base of any container is soft but firm.

The quickest way to deal with an aggressive cat is to drop a coat or towel over it, pick it up wrapped in the towel and pop it into a container, towel and all. It is always advisable to cover a cat with a coat, rug or towel before trying to lift it, even if it appears docile. With really angry or frightened cats you might have to use cat-grab tongs but in many cases you can catch it up by the scruff of the neck, when it should not be able to bite or scratch you. Of course you should not take it by the scruff if it has a spinal injury or the neck is injured.

Sick or injured cats act like many wild animals. Their prime instinct is to escape to a safe place and if an injured cat is still out in the open you need to act fast to catch it safely before it vanishes. Throw a coat over the cat and immediately wedge it between your thighs, bearing down on it as described above, then shout for help. If you are too late, the cat will have crawled away to hide under something, perhaps a shed or a vehicle, and it will certainly not come out when called. It might be necessary to hook it out gently with a crook, or use a grasper to lift it up and swing it into a basket: do not try using your hands to unearth a cat.

An unconscious cat should not be moved but if it is in the middle of the road it will have to be taken to safety. Spread out a coat, put your hands under the animal and slide it carefully on the coat as a stretcher.

Feral cats are much more of a handful than house pets. A stray can be instantly distinguished from a pet cat by its filthy, matted, flea-ridden coat. It will probably have suffered from diarrhoea from eating unsuitable food scraps and its backside and "trousers" might be mucky.

A stray is likely to be used to being kicked and sworn at and unused to handling, and could therefore be vicious and resentful. Treat all strays and ferals with great respect: you must use a grasper for your own safety. If you are "lucky" enough to come across the native wild cat, the personal risk is even greater and you really must get professional help.

All cats, including domestic pets, are highly susceptible to shock and can die of it even if otherwise unharmed. Always treat a cat for shock after any stressful incident by keeping it in a warm, dark, quiet place to recover.

Cattle

If you are inexperienced with cattle, it would be wise to get help; and if theanimal is a bull, on no account should you try and handle it unless you know what you are doing. Be aware that a bull has a flight space around him of about 6 yards and if you invade that space you might not know what has hit you. Most bulls wear nose rings, and you can use a crook through the ring to control the animal: if necessary, give it a little twist to remind him who is in control. Never trust any bull, however well you know him.

Cattle by their very size and weight can unwittingly damage you—perhaps by treading on your foot, or giving you a playful butt. A cow on her own will respond like most animals to firm but gentle and friendly handling, and will relish a good scratch behind her poll or along her back; she will also probably be amenable to halters and tethers, especially if she is a house cow. But most cattle will need to be physically restrained for any kind of treatment, and the equipment needs to be very sturdy.

Cattle are herd animals and hate to be in isolation. They are quite easy to shepherd but often you will be more successful if you amble ahead of them so that they follow you out of curiosity, especially if you are carrying food and call them as you proceed. A dog can be a useful if unwilling lure, too: all cattle like to chase a dog, and if the dog takes them in the right direction, then that is fine.

To persuade an "ornery" cow into a place she has no intention of entering, give weight to the person who is halter-leading her by having two people behind the cow linking hands against her rump and heaving her forward. To keep a cow from fidgeting while she is under treatment for minor injuries etc., hold the tail near the base and lift it up towards the vertical: it will effectively immobilise her.

Deer

There are six species of deer found in the wild in Britain, two of them indigenous (red and roe) and four which have been introduced and have become feral (fallow, sika, muntjac, water deer). Deer are also farmed to an increasing extent, and these are mainly red deer, which are the largest species in Britain. On the whole, the smaller the species the more nervous it is of man: the order of size after the red is fallow, sika, roe, water deer and, smallest of all, muntjac. Males of all these species, except the water deer, have antlers; the water deer and the muntjac have "tusks", or overgrown upper canine teeth.

All deer panic easily, whatever their size, and you must be slow, quiet, positive and confident when handling them, even if they are farmed or park deer reasonably used to humans. They all have acute senses of hearing and smell, and they can all move at high speed. They also have very vulnerable legs which seem to break readily, especially if the deer does panic. All deer are best handled in subdued light: like so many other animals they calm down in darkness, and a blindfold works wonders. Conversely, you can immobilise a deer at night by shining a strong torch beam in its eyes—and this is precisely why some deer are the victims of road traffic accidents. Like most nocturnal creatures, they can be dazzled and disorientated by vehicles' headlights and it takes some time for their eyes to adjust to the glare.

The big red, especially the males during the rut, do sometimes attack people as opposed to instinctive self-defence when cornered, but any male of any deer species can be dangerous in the rut and should be treated with great respect. On the whole, males attack with their heads and antlers but females strike with their feet and their sharp hooves can cause quite a lot of damage. To avoid being boxed in the face, just step back a pace as she strikes. Fallow have a trick of jumping at you from a standing start and landing their cutting hooves on your head or shoulders. Watch out, too, for the back legs: some deer will lash out with a swift series of kicks. A sika might also try and bite, and the tusks of the two smallest species are sharp enough to cause injury, even accidentally.

FIG. 14   DEER THREAT STANCES
Normal alert stance.
Threat stance (1): ears back, neck stretching forward, chin and muzzle lifted, foreleg raised.
Threat stance (2): beginning to rear up. Next stage will be full threat: standing upright on hindlegs ready to strike with forefeet.

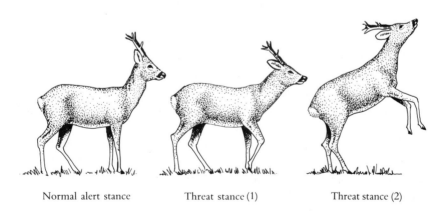

| Normal alert stance | Threat stance (1) | Threat stance (2) |

Keep an eye out for a deer's threat stances (see Fig. 14). For example, the first sign of trouble with a red deer will be a drawing back of the ears, rather like an irritable horse, with a lifting of the muzzle to a horizontal position.

Then a foreleg will be raised, and the next you know the animal is beginning to rear up on its hind legs ready for the boxing match. If a deer is going to bite you, it will tilt its head, snarl its upper lip, grind its teeth, stick out its tongue, show the whites of its eyes and hiss at you. A fully-antlered red stag in the rut, incidentally, is quite capable of disembowelling you, and a hand-reared male of any species is probably the most dangerous of all as it has lost its fear of humans.

In general, uninjured deer should be gradually shepherded into an enclosure, though even fairly generous enclosures can cause great stress. Most adult deer will find any kind of building very claustrophobic, even if it is darkened. Never try putting a roe in such close confinement: it will be shocked to death. And Chinese water deer in any kind of housing will run about nervously and are in danger of overheating themselves.

Injured or sick deer are of course even more likely to succumb to the stress of handling or confinement. Bear in mind that a sick deer can be just as dangerous, even if it appears to be rather quiet. The dilemma is that in order to protect yourself and to protect the animal from injuring itself in its panic, you do need to restrain it, especially by hobbling its legs. You also need to render its antlers less harmful: for example, you could wrap them in sacking or pop a piece of hosepipe over a young roe buck's "pricket" spikes. If a male is "in velvet" his antlers will be sensitive and need protecting with padding.

An injured red stag needs to be brought into a prone position with its antlers (in season) roped at the base, with the other end of the rope tied to something solid like a tree or vehicle, and its front feet loosely hobbled so that it cannot stand up again. It should then be blindfolded before any attempt is made to give first aid, and it is important that the vet should attend on site and tranquillise it before transporting it. If it has already shed its antlers, or if it is a red hind, use a pillow-case over the head as a blindfold (making sure there are breathing holes). With any other deer, remembering that the smaller the species the more timid it is likely to be and the more quietly and gently it needs to be handled, do try and keep the animal prone with its head on the ground and cover it with a blanket, or at least cover its head with a coat, then hobble the legs loosely, unless they are injured. Use a blanket stretcher to move most deer (preferably after sedation): it will probably need four people to lift a red deer but two could manage a roe, and a muntjac can be carried very carefully in a sack. The red will need something the size of a 15 cwt van or a horse trailer for transport but a roe could be slipped into the back of an ordinary van. The little muntjac needs exceptionally quiet, gentle, patient handling: it is more than likely to die of shock from handling and will jerk about all over the place when it is alarmed.

If you have no experience of deer, do please contact an expert to handle a distressed animal. The police, the RSPCA and NARA will either help you themselves or find the right person for you. It is so easy to do more harm than good with a deer.

Dogs

With many dogs, the best approach is the usual quiet, kind and reassuring one. Talk calmly to it, approach steadily but slowly, and you will probably be able to restrain it with no more than a gentle hand. If you can find someone whom the animal knows, your task will be that much easier.

Dogs are frequently the victims of road traffic accidents (RTAs), mostly thanks to irresponsible owners who let them wander. If the animal is not severely injured, muzzle it if necessary (even a friendly dog could bite if it is in pain) and use a collar or lead just in case it decides to make a bolt. A small dog is best transported on someone's lap if the injuries are not serious, and a larger one can go on the back seat of a car, with the lead attached to a fixed point as security against panic or attempted escape.

If a friendly approach fails, you will need to slip some kind of restraint around the dog's neck—a check chain or an improvisation which is free-running so that pressure can be applied or released quickly. The clanking of a chain will frighten an animal who is not familiar with it: leather is kinder. More difficult cases need to be handled with a grasper or even a net.

The more severe the injury, the more likely it is that the dog will react aggressively, and this response will probably be greatest if the animal has a fractured spine, which causes excruciating pain and will probably paralyse its back legs. The agony will provoke it to behave quite abnormally and savagely. It is important to restrain such a dog in order to prevent it attacking people and other animals. You will need to use a grasper to persuade the dog into a prone position; then muzzle it and use a blanket stretcher to take it very carefully into a vehicle for transport.

In the case of a mad dog, your aim is to isolate and confine it, calm it down and get veterinary help as quickly as possible. Be very careful: do not approach the dog but crouch down at a distance that it will not find threatening. Keep your eyes downcast and talk very quietly to reassure it. Keep any movements very slow and smooth. If it begins to approach you out of curiosity, let it come in its own time. Do not rush anything. Slowly slip a collar on it when you can do so without causing alarm. It is almost bound to need a sedative and you should bring the vet to the dog rather than try and take the dog to the surgery.

Body language is the essence of communication with dogs and you should be as alert to the animal's signals as it will be to yours. If you don't like dogs, get someone else to handle the situation.

Ferrets

Ferrets have been domesticated for a very long time indeed, and most are used to being handled and docile with those who understand them. But bear in mind that ferrets are carnivores and can be expert killers. Their instinct is to go for anything remotely resembling say, a mouse, and as their eyesight is very poor they can readily mistake a hesitant finger for such a prey. Their reactions are lightning fast and their bite is both painful and persistent: like their larger relatives, the badger and otter, they tend to lock on and the grip can be difficult to shake. If that happens to you, one of the first solutions is to let the animal's feet rest on the ground rather than dangling in mid-air: it will probably be so relieved to be back on land that it will let go. Sometimes, though, it takes a lot more than that to detach a persistent ferret: you could try pinching the skin on its forehead, or pinching a foot to distract it (but watch out it doesn't instantly flash its teeth into the pinching hand instead!). In dire straits, but only if you are desperate, press your finger against its windpipe or dunk it in a bucket of water so that it has to let go to breathe.

Most ferrets, however, are as easily handled as any pet. You can probably just slip a hand under its body to lift it, or you can grasp (but not grip) it around the shoulders from above, in which case you should support the rear end of its long body as well, especially if it is pregnant or overweight (see Fig. 15). If you put your thumb under its chin, it will not be able to bite you. With a really aggressive animal, which is rare, distract it by wiggling your fingers (at a safe distance) with one hand, then use your other hand to grasp it quickly around the neck and shoulders.

Ferrets are by nature playful and full of unlimited curiosity, especially for anything down a dark hole. To catch an escaped ferret (which is usually lost rather than playing truant), try the tube trick. Ferrets love nothing better than exploring something that looks promisingly like a burrow, so place a good length of drainpipe in the area and let it lead to a box or cage.

Foxes

A fox is more likely to snap and then run away if it can, rather than attack you or clamp on like a badger. It is very easy to get to like foxes, but they are wild animals, not domesticated dogs, and their experience of humans over the centuries has been adverse to say the least. They are therefore unlikely to welcome your attentions, however much you want to help.

Like other underground animals, the fox's urge will be to hide away if it is injured or sick. If you find it out in the open, then it must be in quite a bad way. Use its hiding instinct to lure it into a portable "den" as you would with a badger—say a tea-chest on its side with the entrance largely covered by a cloth. You can "herd" a fox towards the chest in much the same way as you would a pig, using a board in each hand to guide it. Once inside a dark container, it will feel safe.

Do wear gloves to deal with adult foxes, and keep your face away from teeth and claws. Like many animals, foxes sometimes go for the eyes of an enemy.

If the animal is at all active you will probably need to use a grasper or net, or you might try a live-trap of some kind. Once a fox is rolled up in a net or inside a sack, it is quite easy to manage, but it is still advisable to muzzle the animal unless its jaw is injured. (Jaw fractures are quite a common result of RTAs.) To get a muzzled fox into a sack, make a fist-sized hole at the sealed end of the sack, put your hand through it and pull the fox in rump first, then tie the top of the sack. To make sure the fox cannot remove its muzzle, bind its front legs if they are not injured. The bagged fox can then be transported quite safely on the back seat of a vehicle.

If you have no handling tools and the fox is perhaps trapped or too injured to move away, put a good glove on one hand and move it slowly towards the fox so that it can see it clearly. The animal will take a glancing snap at the hand: quickly take the scruff of its neck in your other (bare) hand. In most cases, a firm grip on the scruff is enough to make a fox give up the idea of struggling; perhaps it is reminiscent of maternal control in cubhood.

Goats

Goats can be a bit of a handful: they are often unpredictable and skittish, especially with people they do not know or people who are not familiar with the ways of goats. A billy with horns can also be pretty dangerous and is quite capable of doing damage to your thigh bones or pelvis if he is of an aggressive nature. Always stand *behind* the head.

All goats are agile and can be difficult to confine or restrain. They are excellent jumpers and climbers, and they can also dig their way out under a fence. They tend to turn and face an attacker rather than to flee. They are also full of curiosity, and that is something to be exploited when you want to catch a goat. Walk away, and it will probably follow you.

They are often easier to handle on unfamiliar territory, where they feel confused, but they are extremely nervous of narrow passages like handling races. Domesticated nannies should be well used to handling, however, and will be as tame as any pet, but ferals tend to avoid humans as far as possible.

Guinea-Pigs, Gerbils and Hamsters

For the sake of convenience, this section includes all sorts of small, furry pets
for children irrespective of the family to which they belong.

Chinchillas are usually very gentle creatures which rarely bite, but they do
need gentle handling to avoid leaving fur-bare patches. Hold them very
carefully around the shoulders, or take the base of the tail in one hand and
give them under-body support.

Chipmunks are very different: they object, violently, to being handled and
will probably bite—and bite hard. A tame one can be held in cupped hands,
or by its large neck scruff. A resolutely elusive chipmunk might need to be
caught up in a light butterfly net but do not chase it around the place: the
stress will be too great for it.

Gerbils, like chinchillas, are friendly little things and rarely bite. Hold them
in the palm of your hand but restrain them from leaping off (which they will
try) by holding at the base of the tail. Never hold the end of the tail because
the skin will probably shed. If extra control is needed, wrap the animal in
a cloth or hold it down by the scruff over its shoulders and neck, and it will
become quite relaxed. Quite a few creatures relax under a firm hold from
above: it is the first step towards the tonic immobility in the clutches of a
predator, described earlier.

Guinea-pigs are usually friendly enough and easy to handle, but if frightened
they move at high speed. They can be picked up with one hand around the
shoulders and the other supporting their hindquarters.

Hamsters—beware! They can bite, and the bite is painful. Like ferrets,
they are particularly fond of attacking pointing fingers, but they can usually
be picked up in a cupped hand, or restrained by the scruff of the neck.
Pregnant females or any animal just waking up are more likely to bite than
most.

Hares and Rabbits

Frightened rabbits have several ways of retaliating if you try and handle them:
they might scream, which is unnerving; or bite and scratch, which is painful;
or struggle so hard that they damage their own spines and succumb to
permanent paralysis; or suffer a heart attack under severe stress and fear. With
that catalogue of calamities, it can be seen that careful, quiet handling is
essential. Your aim, of course, is to calm the terrified animal, so often one
of nature's victims in the wild.

A domesticated rabbit can usually be picked up by the scruff of the neck,
with your hand under its rump to support the bodyweight (see Fig. 16). If
you insist on lifting by the ears, that back-end support is even more essential.

Some domestics will resent even a scruff hold and are better with a hand under the chest, so that your thumb and two fingers can hold each foreleg separately.

Any rabbit, tame or wild, which struggles or squeals should really be put down immediately to avoid damage. Try and get the animal into somewhere dark like a sack or strong box, and that should calm it down. Such a container is also good for transporting either rabbits or hares but a wooden box is better, with adequate ventilation holes because these animals do seem to die easily from becoming overheated. Hares can be handled as rabbits but their back-leg kick is even more vigorous and painful, as are their bites.

A loose animal can be lured into a cage live-trap baited with chopped root vegetables, or at worst rabbits can be caught in purse-nets or long-nets (6.5 cm mesh size for adults, 4 cm for youngsters), in which case you will need to hold them by the back legs while you try and disentangle them. They do have the trick of seeming to become acquiescent in the meantime, only to burst suddenly into life and escape at the slightest opportunity.

The disease myxomatosis is only harmful to rabbits: it offers no danger to people or to other animals except for pet bunnies. There is still no cure for it and on no account should you take an infected rabbit into another area and thus spread the disease.

Hedgehogs

You will not have many problems catching up with a hedgehog: its immediate reaction is to roll into a ball and protect itself passively with its spines. The spines might give you a stinging sensation like nettlerash, so wear some gloves if you want to pick the animal up. If you do not have a very thick pair of gloves handy, spread out a handkerchief or piece of newspaper and gently roll the animal on to it so that you can pick it up in a "sling". The hedgehog will obligingly remain rolled up while you transport it.

Then comes the problem of unrolling the animal in order to examine or treat it. Everybody has their own methods. If it is familiar with you, your aim would be to dissuade it from rolling up in the first place and with luck, if you approach it slowly with soothing words and offer your hand for it to sniff, it will accept your presence and allow you to slide your palm very slowly under its stomach and gently lift it up. That is a sign of its confidence in you: it would never stay unrolled for a stranger.

Les Stocker offers several unrolling suggestions in his enjoyable and comprehensive book *The Complete Hedgehog* (which is essential reading for anyone who ever has to handle hedgehogs). One of his ideas is to lift the spiny ball in the palm of your hand from underneath, then rock it gently back and forth: the hedgehog begins to get a little giddy and unrolls to see what on earth is going on. Another trick is to relax the animal by stroking its spines from head to tail, gradually stroking the spines back from the head. Stroking the spines over the rump quite firmly also persuades a hedgehog to uncurl: it tends to lift its head to investigate. Or try Martin Gregory's technique from the *Manual of Exotic Pets:* hold the hedgehog head downwards (if you can work out where its head is!) over a table. It will probably start to unroll cautiously and try to reach the table-top, giving you a chance to take a gentle hold on its hind legs. Or you could try putting it on its rolled-up back and very gently work one stick under its head and another under its hind legs so that it is gradually uncurled, but that is rather undignified, and all animals should be allowed to retain their dignity. Make quite sure there are no loud or sudden noises, or the hedgehog will promptly roll up again.

Hedgehogs are always worth rescuing, and they generally make very good patients, with a high rate of success compared to other wild animals. They can recover from quite appalling injuries.

Horses, Ponies, Donkeys and Mules

As with any other animal, all the equine species respond to firm but gentle and kind handling. Watch a horse's ears for a sure indication of its mood and intent; keep your feet out from under its hooves, and your body well away from a possible kick by a rear leg which could knock you into the ditch or a bite from teeth strong enough to earn your enduring respect. The wound is more than likely to become infected as well as to hurt a great deal, and if there is any likelihood of it biting the animal should be muzzled.

A frightened animal will show symptoms like sweating, shivering and rolled eyes; its first instinct is to bolt, especially back to a familiar environment (in a panic it will even gallop back into its burning stable for security). If it cannot flee, it will rear, buck, bite and kick.

A horse is usually restrained by means of a head collar, halter or bridle (see Fig. 13 for a makeshift horse halter), and if further restraint proves necessary it can be loosely hobbled or have one leg held or tied up. If you need to attend to the rear end of the animal for first aid, have someone pick up the forefoot which is on the same side as that where treatment is needed: this will unbalance the horse and dissuade it from kicking or moving about restlessly. In extreme situations it might be necessary to "cast" a horse, in the manner of cattle, by using carefully placed ropes to urge it into a prone position but this should only be done with professional help.

To calm a restrained horse, try talking quietly into its ears while stroking its muzzle. If it is very restless, a blindfold or a pair of blinkers will help to quieten it. If it has to be led from the light into a dark area, it will need time to adjust its vision.

If you need to handle the animal's legs and feet, do this last—after you have run your hand along its back and belly so that it has due warning of your intentions.

Horses have many blind spots and if you come up unexpectedly you will cause considerable stress. Approach a strange horse as if aiming for its shoulder: it will be able to see you more clearly than from a head-on approach.

Donkeys and mules are much less jumpy than horses; indeed they like to take life at a slow, steady pace and you should fall into a similar frame of mind when handling them. They are very responsive to kindness and consideration, and should always be given plenty of time.

Mink

Mink are mustelids, in the same family as weasels, stoats, polecats and ferrets. Like their wild relatives, they are fearless animals and would not hesitate to give a very good account of themselves if they felt threatened, whatever the size of their opponent. As their bite is vicious and dangerous they should never be handled without very thick, strong gloves. To hold a mink, put one hand around its neck and shoulders, with a thumb under its chin, and the other hand around its hindquarters. It would be preferable to live-trap it in a solid container or, if it is disabled, wrap it up in netting so that a vet can administer a sedative before further inspection and treatment.

Moles

Moles are not happy in captivity, and they frequently die of shock during the first twenty-four hours. However, it *is* possible to live-trap them, or to flick them out of a shallow run by noting their progress and quickly cutting off their rear retreat with a spade, then flicking them out with it.

To hold a mole, take a grip on the loose skin over its back. It can be lifted by its tail but should only be held thus for a very short while, even if you have the other hand over its back with your fingers round its body. It has remarkably powerful front legs and chest muscles, and can dig its way out of all but the strongest containers.

It is rare to see a mole above ground unless it has been killed, and it is even more rare for an injured mole to be treated successfully.

Otters

Otters can be almost as dangerous to handle as badgers if they are frightened or trapped. It is essential to wear thick gloves or to roll them in a net. Like the badger, an otter has a self-locking jaw. It might be possible to escape from its vice-like grip if you snap a dry stick so that it sounds like a bone breaking: with luck, the otter will relax its hold momentarily so that you can remove your poor hand.

The otter is a very brave animal and you need a combination of courage, strength and patience to handle it. It is also very supple, so that it is almost impossible to get a really safe hold on that twisting body. You could try and tangle it up in heavy netting so that a vet can anaesthetise it for inspection and treatment, but keep your hands well out of the way of teeth and claws. Unless you can call up an expert handler, perhaps from the Otter Trust, your best chance is probably the use of *two* graspers: one person uses a grasper at the front end—not just round the neck (it will easily slip the noose off) but round the body behind the front legs. The other person's grasper tackles the rear end simultaneously, then you both apply firm pressure in opposite directions to make sure the animal cannot twist free or double up. Get it into a sack as quickly as possible, or into a large and sturdy box (metal or wood) with a secure lid. Whatever container is used during transport, the otter's environment should be dark and quiet. And, like so many animals, an otter will be much calmer once it *is* in the dark container.

Otters are well protected by the law and any injured or diseased otter should be reported to the police and the NCC.

Pigs

Get experienced help if you have to deal with a pig: the adults can be quite dangerous, and some of them are big enough to do you damage even if they harbour no grudge. A sow with a litter to protect is probably the most dangerous of all: never turn your back on her, or on an injured pig.

Pigs are very intelligent and have acute senses. They do not like strangers but it is possible to make friends with them if you know how. They enjoy a quiet conversation and appreciate any softly spoken sound.

Piglets can bite, but their most usual reaction to being handled is to let out deafening squeals which sound as though they are being slaughtered. Never pick up a piglet unless you are quite certain the sow is securely restrained.

Pigs are home-lovers and do not like being moved. In particular they dislike being shifted from the comfort of a dark pen out into the light, and will quite easily panic. In the open they will scatter and crouch in the undergrowth, or race back to their den, but they are not flock animals like sheep. Treat each pig as an individual if you want to shepherd it: do not abuse or punish it, do not attempt to rush it, but use a board to coax it in the right direction.

Pigs tend to assume that if they cannot see through something they cannot barge through it either which, in view of their size, weight and strength, is a misconception. They go more cheerfully along the level or up a ramp rather than down one and can usually be moved forward if you make a sort of "choo choo" noise. If a pig breaks back, make your "choo choo" sharper and accompany it with sharp hand-claps. A very awkward pig should have a plastic bucket put over its nose and eyes, and it can then be reversed to its destination.

Injured pigs are very difficult to handle. Keep some kind of shield to hand, and get the pig isolated in a confined space. Then get a vet as soon as you can: it is almost impossible to treat an injured pig unless it is unconscious. If you can do so without being savaged, restrain the pig by means of a noose round its upper jaw, passing behind the canine teeth (see Fig. 6).

Pine Martens, Polecats, Stoats and Weasels

The martens (pine, beech, sable etc.) are agile mustelids with longer muzzles and more teeth than the others mentioned in this group; in fact, they are bigger in all respects, and very beautiful if you are lucky enough to see them.

All the animals in this group are highly courageous, like mink, and will bite and clamp, and often give off a pungent and lingering stink for good measure. They are also as supple as otters: you will need to wear stout gloves and to take a grip on them quickly and firmly, with a hand around the neck and forequarters. Pop them into a sack for a short journey, or into a cat-basket or secure wooden box for a longer one—and bear in mind that all mustelids (including ferrets) can escape through unbelievably small holes. You might be able to catch an elusive little weasel with a bird-catching net, or use a live-trap cage or a tunnel, ferret-style.

Like otters, pine martens are protected in law and you should report any find of an injured or diseased marten to the NCC.

Rats, Mice and Voles

If you are lucky enough to find a dormouse, you will find it most amenable: it will not bite and will positively like being handled. Tame rats and mice can be held by the scruff of the neck or the loose skin on their backs or round the shoulders (see Fig. 17), but wild rodents are almost sure to bite in self-defence. The bite of a rat in particular is likely to become infected and can be highly dangerous, passing on such diseases as Weill's disease (leptospiral jaundice) and salmonella poisoning. An aggressive mouse should not be picked up by the scruff of the neck: it will panic. Instead, take it by the base of the tail, but briefly.

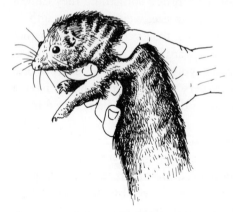

FIG. 15   RESTRAINING A FERRET
Place thumb and forefinger around neck, but do not grip tightly. Keep forelegs between first and second fingers.

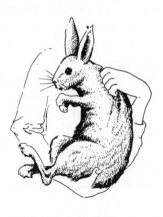

FIG. 16   HOLDING A TAME RABBIT
Take scruff (not ears) in one hand. Hold animal close to your body, supporting weight with other hand under rump.

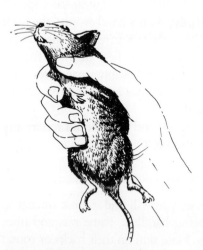

FIG. 17   RESTRAINING A PET RAT
Pick up with hand round shoulders, keeping thumb under chin to prevent biting.

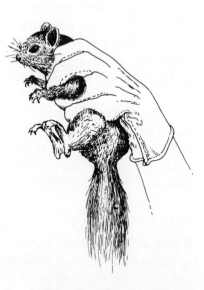

FIG. 18   RESTRAINING A FAMILIAR SQUIRREL
Wear gloves as bites can be severe. Place thumb and finger round neck, front legs between second and third fingers; support weight under armpits. Keep firm hold but do *not* squeeze.

A small rodent can sometimes be trapped under a jam jar, or a rat can have a coat thrown over it and will prefer to remain safely underneath it in the dark than come out again. All the rodents seek to escape and hide. Little ones can be transported in the jam jar if you give them some bedding (for example, shredded paper) and punch some air-holes in the lid; a rat could be picked up along with the coat and bundled, coat and all, into a sack. Use thick gloves when dealing with a rat, but if you get it into a strong bag made of dark, loosely-woven cloth (for air) it will stay in it quietly and probably won't bother to try and chew its way out.

Live-trapping depends on the species. Rats are very wary of anything new, whereas mice are exceptionally inquisitive and will investigate. To remove a rat from a live-trap, stretch the dark-cloth bag over the exit: the rat will gladly run towards the darkness of the bag, the mouth of which can then be secured with an elastic band. To remove a mouse from a live-trap or container, put your cupped hand over the animal and then pick it up by the tail and transfer it quickly to a cage (if you suspend it by the tail for more than a few seconds it will climb up its own tail and bite you). Or offer a mouse access to the kind of wooden boxes that are used for sending 3-inch by 1-inch specimen tubes through the post: it will readily enter one of the holes and sit there with its tail hanging out.

A reasonably docile mouse can be lifted from its container by the tail and allowed to put its front feet on a rough surface. It will automatically try and pull away from you, giving you the chance to take its scruff with the other hand so that you can lift it up for inspection, with your third and fourth fingers of the same hand around the base of its tail.

A tame rat will only bite if it is in pain or frightened; otherwise you should be able to hold it quite easily with your hand round its shoulders and a thumb under its chin just in case it does try to bite. Hold it firmly but not too tightly: it will panic if it feels stifled.

Shrews, which are not rodents but insectivores (like moles, bats and hedgehogs), are handled as if they were rodents but you will need gloves for a water shrew because any bite it gives you is likely to become infected.

Seals

The handling of seals is always best left to the experts. If you find an injured or distressed seal, contact your nearest seal sanctuary (for example, in Norfolk, Cornwall, Skegness, Oban and Cardigan) or marine life centre, or the Sea Mammal Research Unit in Cambridge, or the RSPCA/SSPCA. In the meantime, keep people in general and dogs in particular well away from the animal: give it as much peace as possible while you wait for assistance.

If the seal is a young pup which seems to have been abandoned on a beach or sandbank but has no apparent injury—**leave it alone!** Do *not* handle it; do not even go anywhere near it—you might be passing between the pup and its mother, who is probably watching from the sea and will promptly desert it for real. On no account try and return it to the sea: a young pup does not live in the water all the time and will probably not be strong enough to do so anyway, so that the outcome will be sheer exhaustion. *Please* listen to the advice of seal experts and do not fool yourself that you "know better".

If you are all alone on an island with no means of contacting an expert, so that you must yourself handle a seal which is definitely in trouble, bear in mind that seals do bite. Even a young one will bite in self-defence. An adult's bite can be severe enough to cripple you and is very likely to become infected. Be particularly careful with the grey seal, a bigger animal than the common seal and much less amenable. Approach from the rear and, for safety's sake, only hold it by the tail flippers if it needs to be handled at all. An adult could be carefully hauled up a smooth ramp into a means of transport, preferably with a groundsheet or something similar underneath it on which it can be dragged. A pup can be transported in a shallow box: it will not try and jump out.

Sheep

Sheep are defenceless and therefore vigilant animals who find safety in tight flocking. Isolation terrifies them. They like to be at least four or five in number, and are much easier to handle if the minimum grouping is borne in mind: three sheep are just about impossible to manage. They are very "visual" and like to see what is going on around them, and they react very quickly to danger. Sheep are susceptible to panic, and their immediate reaction is to flee, preferably uphill or towards the light. When being shepherded, they do like to see an opening ahead of them, even if it is only an illusion, and they are very loth to enter a dark place, nor do they like walking into their own shadows or going into water. They have a strong urge to follow a moving sheep ahead of them.

If you find sheep wandering on a road, persuade them into the nearest field and notify the police, or of course the local farmer if you know him. Shepherd them calmly: if you start to run around in a panic, so will they—and that could kill them on a hot day. The best attitude with sheep is quiet authority, especially if they are already distressed, and you should keep all your movements calm and your voice low.

If an injured or shocked sheep is already lying down, keep it that way, because if you let it find its feet it will flee. You might need to kneel firmly, but gently, on its neck to keep its head down and reduce struggling, but you should try and give it a cushion under the head. It might be necessary to bind its hind legs together to prevent them flailing about. An RTA casualty will probably need no restraint and can be given first aid and then carried on a blanket stretcher to a place of safety for treatment.

When a flock has suffered the trauma of savaging by a dog on the rampage, the animals will be so shocked that they will be much easier to handle, even those which have not been injured. Many of the injuries will be horrific and the vet needs to be summoned immediately. You will also need plenty of help as you want to try first to isolate the uninjured sheep in a corner of the field. If there are other people nearby ask someone to stand with them to keep them quiet (in their shocked state they will be easy to control) while you begin to attend to the casualties.

Sheep also have a habit of getting themselves entangled in fencing mesh or bramble thickets, and the more they struggle in a thicket the more their fleece gets twisted into the undergrowth. You will need to use your knees to grip the sheep around its body just in front of its back legs, approaching the animal from behind, then grab the neck fleece behind the head with one hand while you use the other to try and untangle everything.

Another problem, especially with the rather sturdy downland sheep like the Southdown, is that the sheep somehow gets itself on its back and cannot roll back on its feet. It is essential to turn it the right way up because it will get acute indigestion and could even die. Downland breeds of sheep tend to be more amenable than most and you will find it quite easy to kneel by the animal and reach over to grab a hold of the fleece on its back and roll it over.

To catch a sheep, approach from behind (they have a blind spot behind the head when the head is raised). Getting a sheep into a docile position sitting on its hams is known as "casting", for which there are a number of methods. Put one hand on its muzzle and turn its head back along its side so that it faces to the rear. The sheep will slowly collapse to the floor. Quickly grab hold of both its front legs with both hands and tilt it so that it sits on its backside at about sixty degrees from upright. In that position, it will relax. For a smaller breed you should still approach from behind but you can just grab it round the neck with one hand and quickly lift up its front end, then walk the animal backwards until it plumps down on its rump. Gently! A further method for smaller breeds is shown in Fig. 19.

To lift a sheep over an obstacle like a wall or fence, or into a trailer, catch it from behind as just explained and get it standing on its hind legs between your knees. Stand with your left side to the obstacle and have your left arm round the sheep's neck and use your left hand to hold its right front fetlock near its neck (see Fig. 20). Grip the fleece along its right side with your right hand then use your knee to lever the animal up to the top of the obstacle leaning back towards you so that it is virtually lying on its back on the top, then let it roll over to land on its feet on the other side.

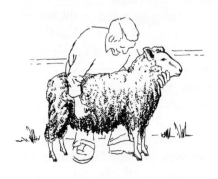

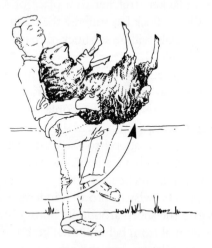

FIG. 19 "CASTING" A SHEEP
For a fairly light sheep. Place left hand under its chin and stand close with your knees bent. Right hand holds wool and loose skin on flank, lifting right hind leg off the ground, simultaneously nudging animal with your knees to prevent bracing. Gently turn animal to sit on its rump between your feet, with its withers between your knees.

FIG. 20   LIFTING A SHEEP OVER AN OBSTACLE

The shepherd's crook is of course the classic piece of equipment for catching sheep but use it with care if you are hooking an animal by the legs—you do not want to cause bruising. It can also be used to hook an animal by the neck

Squirrels

Squirrels have a most vicious bite and are so quick to react that the bite is almost unavoidable. If you must handle one, use very strong gloves and hold the animal firmly, as shown in Fig. 18 on p. 46 then drop it immediately into a container (it will probably get you even then). They are very agile animals and can easily twist up on themselves to deal with a tail hold. Even an injured squirrel will be impossible to catch if it can bolt up a tree or wall.

Unlike so many other animals, squirrels do *not* like being in an enclosed box. If they must be contained (which they will resent) they would prefer a cage. Any live-trap design should take this preference into account. A container used for transport on a longish journey *must* be of metal: the squirrel's gnawing powers are legendary.

Whales, Dolphins and Porpoises

The main problems with these cetaceans are likely to be connected with stranding and beaching. Methods of dealing with such situations are described in Chapter 4; suffice to say here that expert help is essential and you should immediately contact the local RSPCA/SSPCA, the coastguard, the police, the NCC, and possibly the local fire brigade (who have lifting gear and of course hoses). Above all—urgently—call a veterinary surgeon to assess the animal's state of health before any decisions are taken on the next stage of the rescue. In the meantime, it is important to protect the beached animal by keeping away dogs, bounty hunters and the curious.

HANDLING AMPHIBIANS, REPTILES AND INVERTEBRATES

Some of our native amphibians and reptiles have very special protection in law (see Chapter 10), and if you come across injured specimens of an endangered species you should get advice on how best to handle the situation. Approach the NCC, the RSPCA, your local wildlife hospital or a vet who has suitable experience. An animal like the natterjack toad, for example, is so rare that you virtually have a duty to save it!

Most amphibians and reptiles become less active (and are therefore easier to handle) if you pop them in the fridge for a while. Make sure, however, that the temperature is no lower than about 4 °C: if ice crystals form in their bodies, the pain and distress will be acute. A few minutes' fridge treatment is suitable for water tortoises, lizards, small snakes, newts, frogs and toads—in escape-proof containers, of course! Do *not* use the deep-freeze.

Amphibians

Most amphibians (and the class includes frogs, toads, newts and salamanders) do not like being handled or restrained. Their moist skin is delicate and, if you must handle them, keep your hands slightly damp and also absolutely free of any chemicals, which will be readily absorbed by the amphibian's skin. Some of them produce unfriendly secretions (for example, the toad) and it is wise to wear rubber gloves, especially if you have any open cuts on your hands. Their moist skins are often slippery enough to make holding difficult anyway, and you could use damp towels or soft nets. If the animal needs to be transported, give it moist surroundings by lining a wooden box with damp moss or damp tissues. It is important to avoid desiccation, loss of skin mucus or contact with irritants and toxic substances. Minor wounds can be bathed in a saline solution of common salt (2 per cent) in water.

Most of the amphibians are rather shy and want to get out of your sight, but you might be able to hold a frog or a toad cupped in your hand with its hind legs dangling between your fingers. Some toads eventually become tame enough to welcome hand-feeding, and the slow-moving garden toad can be almost as friendly as the gardener's robin. Great characters, toads! If they cannot escape, they will swell up in an attempt to terrify you with their size, but they cannot harm you. If their bluff does not work, they can become quite distressed and will begin to breathe rather rapidly.

Reptiles

Of Britain's native species of snakes, only the adder is poisonous and its main concern will be to escape from you and hide somewhere. If it cannot, and if it is cornered or suddenly trodden on, then it might bite. Its jaws are not big enough to damage anything more than your fingers or toes, though a young child's limbs might be vulnerable. It is very rare indeed for an adult to die from an adder bite, though there will be considerable discomfort, and the best course of action if a person is bitten is to remain very calm and reassuring, keeping the victim quiet and getting them to a doctor quickly. Nevertheless, non-experts should not attempt to handle adders.

Grass snakes are not poisonous, though they might let off a stinking mess (from both ends!) in the presence of a stranger. That is their only means of self-defence, apart from playing dead (which they can do quite dramatically). Otherwise they are generally amenable animals and are easy to tame.

Non-native snake species should be treated with respect and if you are in any doubt that a snake might be poisonous, leave the handling of it to an expert. If necessary, capture it in a catching net and transfer it immediately into a sack or cotton bag or box.

If a snake is handled too soon after its meal, it will be sick or regurgitate its food: watch out! In principle, do not try and catch up or handle a snake, or a lizard, unless it is obviously injured and able to be helped, or is in danger from, say, road traffic or predators.

To pick up a disabled or nervous non-poisonous native snake, hold it behind its head between your thumb and second finger, with the first finger on top of the head, then lift it with a firm but gentle grasp, with your other hand holding it around the middle of its body to support its weight.

Remember that a slow-worm is not a snake but a lizard and, like other lizards, it should never be grasped by the tail, which will probably be cast off if you do. Slow-worms, as any country child knows, are enchantingly friendly creatures and seem to be quite happy to be handled. To catch a more active lizard, use a catching net if necessary; otherwise a small lizard can often be cupped in your hand, with your first finger under its throat and your thumb lightly resting on the back of its head or neck. A larger exotic can be held round the neck (firmly but gently) with its body tucked under your arm and its tail held in your other hand. Watch out: some of the big lizards have powerfully thrashing tails and scratching claws, which means you will need to wear longish gloves or gauntlets.

Turtles and tortoises are instantly distinguished by their shells, or carapaces. Land tortoises move notoriously slowly and are very easy to catch but will withdraw into their shells if alarmed. They can be induced to poke their heads out again if they are put in a shallow container of tepid water. Water tortoises will probably need to be caught with a net: you could try by hand but their shells tend to be slippery when wet so use a glove or cloth. Some of them do try to bite and it is advisable to hold them by the shell at the back end, with the head away from you, especially if it is a snapping turtle or a long-necked terrapin, both of which can be aggressive and can inflict quite painful bites.

To encourage a soft-shelled turtle to put its head out, turn it on its back so that it has to put out its head in order to try and turn over again. If you find a marine turtle in distress, contact the NCC or your local wildlife hospital for help.

Invertebrates

Like amphibians and reptiles, most invertebrates are more docile if they have been put in the fridge for a while to slow down their metabolism. Thirty minutes is too long, and the temperature should be no less than 4 °C.

Invertebrates can suffer from many different diseases and are especially vulnerable to infectious outbreaks, in which case individuals should be isolated. They also succumb frequently to physical accidents, getting squashed or battered or pecked or de-winged. Many have the ability to regenerate lost limbs. A wounded arthropod (and that includes crustaceans, spiders, millipedes, centipedes, insects etc.) can literally be patched up with glue if it has a hard outer casing which has been damaged.

HANDLING BIRDS

It bears repeating time and again: if you find a fledgling of any species of bird leave it alone unless it is obviously injured or is in danger from predators like cats. The parents are probably close by, waiting for you to disappear so that they can get on with the job of feeding their young. However, if it seems to have fallen out of its nest but is not injured, or if it is obviously at risk from predators, put it out of reach of the latter in the cover of some bushes, as high as possible and near the nest (but not in it) if you know where it is. Or put it in an open box in the shade, protected from the rain and out of predator reach, in a place where the parents can find it. There is more about fledglings and nestlings in Chapter 8.

Garden and Cage Birds

If you find an injured or distressed adult bird which allows you to catch it easily, it probably has major problems but *might* be only stunned from impact with a window, or simply exhausted. A stunned bird which looks groggy will usually recover completely after a while (perhaps as much as an hour) and can be moved to a warm, dark, sheltered, safe spot in the meantime. The same applies to an exhausted bird with no apparent injuries, but if it has not recovered within a few hours it needs expert help.

Any vulnerable bird will be put under worse stress if it has the impression that you are a predator. Avoid swooping down on it from above like a hawk, and certainly do not chase it about: that will almost inevitably lead to the bird's sudden death. Many a wild bird, and many a cage bird too, has been known to die of heart failure under the stress of capture, even if it was initially perfectly healthy. The kindest capture is by dropping a cloth over it so that it is in darkness: nearly all species, except owls, become calmer and feel safer in the dark. However, different ways of handling various larger species are described later in this section.

Small birds of most kinds, up to the size of, say, a duck, and whether wild or cage birds, are much easier to catch in subdued light. If the bird is already confined to a room or shed, make the room dark and then use a torch with a red filter. Wear light gloves or use tissues or a handkerchief when handling the bird to avoid the sweat from your hands damaging the insulation properties of its feathers. Approach slowly, but deliberately.

Cage birds, especially budgerigars and certain parrots, are quite prepared to bite, and a parrot's bite can be dangerous, while even a budgie is inclined to increase its grip on you rather than let go. Smaller wild birds are generally divided into two types: those that eat insects are termed softbills, and those that use their beaks to crack seeds are called hardbills, with'good reason—if a hardbill like a finch takes a nip at you, it will hurt! Some of the corvids, too, should only be handled with good gloves. In an emergency, a double thickness of towel will give you some protection from parrots and most corvids, but watch out for a raven.

Some of the larger birds can be caught with a catching net or by dropping a towel, coat, sweater, shirt or anything else that is handy over them. You could devise an arm's-length box catcher: get a suitable size of cardboard box, give it a length of branch or a broomstick as a handle and trap the bird under the box (see Fig. 21). To get the bird out of these temporary catching devices, remove the catcher or cloth very slowly, keeping its head covered to keep it calm, and try to get your hands round its body so that its wings are in the naturally folded position and cannot flap about. Lower it slowly into a suitable container but support its feet as you do so: if they are left dangling in mid-air the bird will think it is in flight and will start flapping.

To examine a bird for injuries, sit on the floor if it is a small one so that it does not damage itself should it slip from your hand. Put your palm over its back, controlling the wings with your thumb on one side and two fingers on the other, and your first two fingers slightly crooked on either side of its neck as if you were a seam bowler (see Fig. 22). This hold allows you to turn the bird on its back to inspect its underside as well, blowing the feathers apart gently to expose external injuries. Restrain its legs with your little finger if necessary. Be careful not to grip the bird too firmly, especially if it is a small one: it must be able to breathe easily.

Birds which are too big to be held in the palm of one hand should be taken firmly but gently in two, with both your thumbs along the back, so that someone else can examine the bird's underside. Turn it over in a similar hold with your thumbs along the breast for an examination of its back. It would be a kindness to have the bird resting on a cushion. Watch out for a scratch, intentional or otherwise, from its claws. The special handling of oiled birds, birds of prey, waterfowl etc. is described later but it would be wise to slip an elastic band over the beak of something like a crow for your own protection, making sure you do not obstruct its nostrils.

Transport containers for birds can be anything which is big enough to contain them, as long as it gives them enough darkness and privacy for a sense of security, and not so much space that they can flap about and injure themselves but enough for easy breathing. A very small bird could be carried in a paper bag, for example. Something the size of a sparrow, robin or blackbird needs a container about 4½ inches high by 5½ inches wide by 9 inches long. There are some very useful disposable travelling boxes available from those who cater for cage-bird breeders, made of heavy cardboard in various sizes, and there is a big range of commercial carrying boxes ranging from about 6 inches by 12 inches to as big as 6 feet square, in either wood or metal. Suppliers advertise their equipment in specialist journals like *Cage & Aviary Birds*. If you are using some kind of cage, the bird will be under considerable stress unless you can cover most of the cage: the aim is to let the bird feel hidden and also to avoid it being alarmed by movements outside its container. If it can see out, it will try and escape and will injure itself against the cage walls in its panic. Keep it dark, keep it warm, keep it quiet. Improvise with something like a shoe-box or an ice-cream carton for smaller birds, both with air-holes punched in the lid and with some soft material like tissues in the base, but not hay.

Poultry and Gamebirds

Apart from their different reactions to the human race because of domestication or lack of it, gamebirds are similar in many ways to farmyard poultry; indeed, a chicken is a domesticated species of pheasant, and so is a peacock. They all relax in the dark and are much easier to handle in very subdued light.

A chicken can be held in both hands with one on each side so that your thumbs keep the wings from flapping (an imperative for all birds of all species, families and sizes). Or you can slide one hand under its body, from the front, and grasp its legs, with the other hand over the back to take care of the wings, then tuck it in the crook of your arm (see Fig. 23). Something like a turkey is less amenable and much more of a handful: its wings are surprisingly strong and it could bruise your hand with its beak or scratch with its talons.

Gamebirds are very nervous of humans, which in view of their persecution is hardly surprising. The capercaillie is the only one which might be aggressive, though a hen pheasant with a brood of chicks will run at you hissing with her wings flapping and will have a go at your legs with her beak like any other mother hen. If you need to capture an injured gamebird, it is probably a kindness to have several people involved in order to reduce the time to a minimum. A net is very useful if you do not have a reliable soft-mouthed retrieving dog handy. You can either use a typical catching net like a large landing-net or butterfly net, or you could try herding the bird gently into an improvised long-net—perhaps some fruit netting or fish net, or even some tennis net for a larger bird, making sure that the mesh is not large enough for the bird to get its head through and strangle itself. The bird's aim will be to escape from you, and it will make frantic efforts to do so until it is covered by a blackout cloth or bag-net. Its self-defensive pecks and scratches

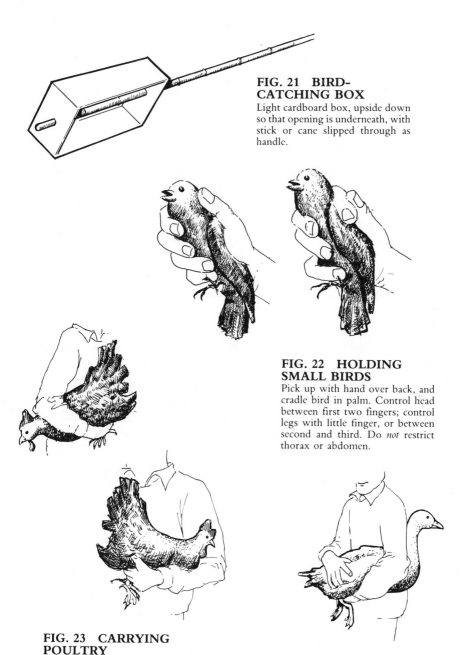

FIG. 21   BIRD-CATCHING BOX
Light cardboard box, upside down so that opening is underneath, with stick or cane slipped through as handle.

FIG. 22   HOLDING SMALL BIRDS
Pick up with hand over back, and cradle bird in palm. Control head between first two fingers; control legs with little finger, or between second and third. Do *not* restrict thorax or abdomen.

FIG. 23   CARRYING POULTRY
Hold legs between fingers. Tip bird's body slightly forwards or rest in crook of arm.

FIG. 24   CARRYING A DOMESTIC DUCK OR GOOSE

are unlikely to be very effective, but you must restrict its wings as soon as possible, and *keep* them restricted. If you put the bird in a box, it should be small enough to prevent wing-flapping damage even if it is dark inside. Many gamebirds have long tails, of course, which can make it awkward to contain them: try a soft zip-up hold-all, leaving the tail protruding through an opening, but make a point of binding or almost trussing the bird first so that it cannot struggle in the bag.

Ducks

Waterfowl respond best to firm but gentle handling, and to warm, dark accommodation. The biggest problem in catching them up is to keep them out of the water. If a bird is already on land, get between it and the water. Do *not* chase it. Sidle towards it slowly without looking in its direction then, when the moment is right, throw a coat over it or a net. If it is on the water and is seriously injured, you will probably have to use a landing-net: it will do its utmost to remain on the water, where it feels safe, and you will only subject it to possibly fatal stress if you attempt to force it on to the land. An injured or frightened duck is likely to dive and remain submerged, which makes it very difficult indeed to catch, and in extreme cases owners of ornamentals who need to transport their elusive diving ducks have been known to drain the pond in order to catch the duck. However, the first trick is to be very patient and try to lure the duck with bread on the water until it is in range of a landing-net. If you miss with the net, it will dive, and you might be able to locate it by the air bubbles so that you can try an underwater scoop. If you miss that, which you will, the bird is likely to sneak under overhanging waterside vegetation and you will need sharp eyes and patience to find it: the camouflage is excellent. Once a duck is wary of you, it is probably best to sit down quietly for a while—quite a long while—and try again later.

Be very careful with the plumage of any water bird. Try and keep your hands off it, especially if there is any sweat. Wrap the bird in clean cloth or sacking to keep the wings secure, but leave the head and neck protruding (you could use a pillowcase) while you carry it to a more suitable container such as a cardboard box for transport (see Fig. 24 on p. 57 for carrying position). Have plenty of newspaper or clean old cloths in the base of the box: ducks are messy squitters at the best of times, and the volume and liquidty of their droppings increases under stress. Do you best to keep the stuff off their plumage.

No water bird should be restrained or confined for a moment longer than necessary.

Swans and Geese

If you find a swan in trouble, contact one of the swan support and rescue groups, who will usually go anywhere at any time to save a swan and who are experts in dealing with their problems. You could also ask for help from the RSPCA or the police, and you will *need* help.

Swans are large birds and should be handled with care. Although stories of them being able to break a man's arm with their wings might be exaggerated, they certainly will beat at you with their wings, which are very large and very powerful. If you can, keep the bird's chest and neck low for your own safety. A knock from a swan's wing will take the skin off your knuckles or your shins, and a goose, though less damaging, could hurt you too. So one of your first aims, for the sake of the bird as well as yourself, is to get those wings under control and bound to its body in the normal resting position (see Fig. 24 on p. 57).

Watch out for beaks, too, especially in this case with a goose, but the damage is more likely to be bruising than anything else. However, the bird could well aim for your face and eyes so keep out of the way, or get the head covered as soon as possible.

If a goose comes at you with apparent aggression, stretching out its neck, hissing, and perhaps spreading its wings, call its bluff and advance rather than retreat. Unless it is protecting a nest, it will turn and run away. That is your opportunity to catch it, from behind, and secure it before it recovers its self-esteem. Both geese and swans can be caught from behind with the aid of a crook: hook it round the neck and twist the tool slightly so that the bird cannot slip free, then draw it towards you firmly until it is within reach. Take the neck in your free hand, drop the crook and force the bird's head towards the ground. Then stand behind the wings, take hold of them where they join the body and lift the bird bodily off the ground if you can. Take your other hand off its neck and put it under the body, then turn yourself so that the bird's rear end can be propelled into an open sack with its wings carefully folded and its feet tucked up. Leave its head protruding from the mouth of the sack, which should be tied around its neck tightly enough to prevent escape but loosely enough for it to breathe easily. Then you can transport it in the back of a vehicle. You might find it much easier to chop a corner off a sack and drop it over the bird, which will be happy to push its head through the hole; then you can tie up the mouth of the sack at the tail end. Sometimes you will be able to carry the bird under your arm, with the other hand holding the neck just behind the head.

There are more elaborate ways of "trussing" the bird for transport to ensure that it does no further damage to itself, especially if you do not happen to have a sack handy. For the sake of the vehicle's driver you need to restrict the bird in some way during transport, perhaps by hobbling its legs if there is no second person to hold it.

Herons, Waders and Rails

These water birds tend to have beaks that could cause varying degrees of damage: keep your face well away from them. The heron and all the waders tend to stab at the eyes, though the smaller ones will be more desperate to escape than attack. It is wise to wrap string, insulating tape or elastic bands around a long, pointed beak for safety, but not for any length of time.

Herons need firm but gentle handling: their bone structure is fragile and rough treatment could result in fractures and internal injuries. Grasp the bird by its neck, just below the head, then tuck the rest of its body under your arm. Hood its eyes with some kind of blindfold and then let it travel loose in the back of a vehicle. It will probably keep quite still if it cannot see. Do not cramp up the legs of any long-legged bird in transport, as there is a strong possibility of inducing paralysis. If one leg is broken, lie the bird on its side with its legs gently stretched out, its wings secured and its head covered. If its beak has been bound for carrying, make sure the binding is removed for the journey in the vehicle.

Coots and moorhens, which can become quite tame in the open, can both bite and scratch if under threat or confined. Their movements are quick and sudden, so do not be taken by surprise. Their claws are to be respected and, as with all birds in this group, their heads should be controlled and you should keep your face well away from beak-reach.

A small wader could be put into a paper bag for transport. It will probably find security more attractive than escape at that stage.

Seabirds

Like inland waterfowl, seabirds feel safer on the water and will make determined efforts to reach it. Get yourself between the bird and the sea, and get other people to help as well. Again like waterfowl, the slow, sideways approach is best, with your eyes averted from the target bird. Use a catching net or throw a coat over it, then remove the coat gradually until you can grasp the bird with a gloved hand just behind its head, using the other to keep its wings close to its body (between your knees if necessary). Keep your face well away from the stabbing beak: for added protection bind it with your handkerchief or an elastic band, making sure the bird can still breathe properly. A bite from a gull, for example, can be more than unpleasant, and a gannet's beak is as effective as a hacksaw. Watch out for the claws, too.

And be prepared for a very noisy protest when the bird is caught.

Transport the bird in a container in which it has enough space to sit comfortably but not so much that it gets thrown around by the movement of a vehicle. The container should be well ventilated but warm, and keep it dark to calm the bird so that it does not struggle.

With oiled birds, the major problem is the ingestion of oil and a darkened container should discourage it from trying to preen and thereby swallow more of the horrible stuff. If the beak was muzzled during capture, it must be unbound for the journey in case the bird vomits from stress. For a bird used to wheeling over the oceans, the trauma of capture and confinement is enormous.

Pigeons

The first reaction to a racing pigeon in the garden should be to leave it alone: it is often down for a drink and will go off again of its own accord when it has rested. However, if it seems to be exhausted and there are predators about, put it somewhere safe. Entice it with corn into a garage, greenhouse or outhouse; close the door to keep out predators but try to provide a way for the pigeon to leave if it wants to. Make sure it has water for drinking and bathing; you could also leave a supply of food (barley, wheat, oats or chicken corn) but if you do feed the bird it might decide it has found a good home. If it is evening, close the bird in for the night and let it out in the morning, when it will probably fly off quite happily.

The pigeon will have a ring on its leg which helps to identify its owner and it might even have its home address stamped on its primary (flight) feathers. Most pigeons are used to being handled, of course, and to pick a bird up hold it round the body, keeping its wings closed. Have its feet side by side between two of your fingers, with your thumb over the primary feathers to retain the wings, and use your other hand under its breast to support its weight. Now you can check the ring number to make contact with the bird's owner who might (or in some cases, unfortunately, might not) be prepared to make arrangements for its return. Note all the details of the number, including letters. For example, NEHU is the North of England Homing Union, SHU is the Scottish Union, IHU the Irish and so on. Then contact the Royal Pigeon Racing Association (RPRA) (see directory in Chapter 11). Be warned that you might be playing host to the pigeon for a week or more while arrangements are made, but with luck there will be a local pigeon fancier willing to take it off your hands in the meantime. The ring also includes a date, which indicates to within five or six days the bird's age— and as long as it is less than ten years old the RPRA will be able to trace the bird's owner even if it has changed hands since birth. The number on the ring is its registration number. Sometimes you will find a bird with a foreign registration but, again, the RPRA can trace the source and advise you on what should be done.

The owner should make all the necessary transport arrangements but sometimes will express total disinterest in the bird or will want you to find a container and "post" it back. The RPRA can provide a proper box (they will post it to you) designed jointly by the RSPCA and British Rail for transporting pigeons by rail or by Interlink. The box looks cramped, but that is on purpose so that the bird cannot turn around or be thrown about: it can travel safely in such confinement for up to twenty-four hours.

Birds of Prey

All birds of prey, whether day-flying raptors or owls, should only be handled with gloves—and heavy, reinforced gloves in most cases. (The gloves will also protect you if the bird is diseased or poisoned.) Their beaks and especially their talons can be dangerous. Their feet are their main weapons and tools, with very sharp, strong, slashing claws and a powerful grip which is quite unshakeable. Indeed, the more you struggle, the more vice-like the grip becomes, and the talons can penetrate right through to the bone. They really do need experienced handling by people who understand them. If you must catch up the bird yourself, do not handle it any more than necessary, then put it in a warm, dark, ventilated box (never a cage) of adequate size until an expert can take charge of it.

Over many centuries of falconry, a good store of knowledge on the handling of all kinds of birds of prey, whether tame or completely wild, has been built up. One of the most useful tips is that a blindfolded bird is a quiet bird. You might not happen to have a falconry hood to hand, but even an old sock slipped over the bird's head should do the trick, as long as you make a hole for its beak so that it can breathe: if it cannot see, it will not bite. But *do not* try hooding an owl.

The "sudden darkness" technique works during capture too: if the bird is unable to fly, throw a coat over it. Then gradually reveal its talons so that you can take a hold on its legs, keeping its head covered so that it stays quiet while you slip the other (gloved!) hand underneath its body so that the bird can be lifted into a container like a cardboard box for transport. Do not use a cat-basket as there are all sorts of jagged snags inside it.

The talons are particularly dangerous when a bird is lying injured. Its first instinct will be to try and hide, and if it cannot it might "play dead", crouched down and rigid with its beak agape pathetically. Do not be fooled, either into assuming that it is in fact dead or into trusting that it is harmless. It *might* remain rigid when you pick it up, but it might suddenly turn on to its back and defend itself with those talons. In that case let it latch on to a strong stick instead of your hand: it will grip as tightly as it would have gripped its prey or your hand, and you can probably lift it, upside down and still hanging on to the stick, so that you can transfer it into a big container (a tea-chest is ideal). Once it is inside, partially close the lid so that the light is subdued. When it can no longer see you, it will probably relax its grip on the stick which you can then remove. With a smaller bird, you could protect yourself by padding its claws with adhesive tape while you apply first aid, but this should be removed as soon as you have finished the treatment and before it is confined for transport.

A diurnal bird of prey can usually be transported with no more restraint than a blindfold—perhaps a handkerchief placed over its head and tied under the beak so that it stays in place (always remembering to leave the nostrils uncovered for breathing). It will probably sit quite happily in the vehicle just like that, though it would be safer to put it in a well ventilated cardboard box.

An injured owl does not need to be hooded for transport. It will only want to hide, and can probably be allowed to travel loose in the vehicle, where it will find itself a dark, safe corner—probably on the floor. If you are trying to catch an owl at night, you can very easily dazzle it into submission with a sudden bright light, and then simply pick it up—it will need about quarter of an hour to adjust its night vision again.

If an owl does get a grip on you with its talons, do not try and pull away. Its instinct will be to tighten its grip on a prey that seems to be trying to escape. If you can bear it, just relax—"play dead"—and wait until the owl releases you of its own accord. An owl usually gives a warning before it strikes: it rears back in preparation. Throw a coat over it, or a sweater or even a scarf, and pick it up all in a bundle.

CHAPTER THREE

FIRST AID

EMERGENCY CHECKLIST

In any emergency situation, the principles of animal rescue are:

- Assess the situation, as calmly and quickly as possible.
- Bear in mind your own safety: you are no good to the animal if you become incapacitated.
- Remove the life threat or cause of pain.
- Carry out resuscitation if needed.
- Relieve immediate pain.
- Prevent further damage or suffering or shock.
- Avoid causing undue stress.
- Only move, handle or confine the animal if essential.
- Attempt limited emergency first aid: get professional help as soon as possible.
- Look after shocked human witnesses as well.

ASSESSMENT

Quick thinking is essential if life is at risk: a few seconds can make all the difference, but beware of making a situation worse by not thinking at all. Be in control of the situation and of yourself; take a deep breath, keep calm, be resolute in your actions and be reassuring to the animal and to other people, especially the owner of a domestic animal or perhaps the driver who has accidentally run over an animal. People need help too. If you feel incapable of dealing with a situation yourself, get someone else who can, but you will be surprised at your own resources in an emergency.

Try not to move an animal before you have more carefully assessed the damage, and try to take the life threat or cause of pain away from the animal rather than vice versa, though obviously in some situations that will be impossible—for example, if the animal is in a burning building or is drowning. Also in the case of, say, heatstroke or poisonous fumes, clearly your aim is to take the animal away from the hot or poisoned environment immediately, but in the case of accidents where internal injury or fractures might have occurred you need to be prepared to give first aid on the spot without moving the casualty until you know more about the extent of the damage.

The indications of major injury might include:

- Loss of consciousness.
- Difficulty in breathing.
- Major bleeding.
- Obvious signs of shock.
- Fractures.
- Inability to stand.
- Obvious pain on movement.

The immediate first-aid steps are to clear the airways and apply artificial respiration if necessary; stop major bleeding; treat for shock.

If the animal is **unconscious** you might have to act quickly to save its life. Do not move it. Get someone to summon immediate veterinary assistance and in the meantime check the following points:

- Is there a pulse or heartbeat? (If there is no sign at all that the heart is working, you will need to apply cardiac massage.)
- Is the animal breathing? (If so, at what rate and depth? If not, give artificial respiration.)
- Is its temperature subnormal? (Feel its extremities.)
- Are its eyes dull? Do they react to stimuli? Are the pupils either dilated, contracted, or of different sizes?
- Is there any unusual colouring of its lips, gums, or the inside edge of its eyelids? Are they very pale (indication of shock or haemorrhage), tinged blue (heart or breathing problems) or yellowish (jaundice or kidney problems)?

- Are there any reflexes at all (eyes, ears, jaw)?

- Are the limbs relaxed (as in shock) or rigid (for example, fits, strychnine poisoning)?

- Is there any bleeding from the ear canals? (This could indicate skull or brain damage, though it might only be damage to the ears themselves.)

- Is there any bleeding from the mouth or nose? Or any evidence of vomiting?

- Are there any indications of injury to the spine (partial or total paralysis) or limbs (fractures, dislocation, deformity, swellings etc.)?

- Are there external signs of other wounds?

Never assume that an animal is dead. It might be stunned or "playing dead"; it might not be "brain dead". Even if it has stopped breathing and there is no pulse, there is still hope—albeit fairly remote in the case of wildlife. If it really is dead, there will be no heartbeat or pulse, no eye reflex, and, essentially, no nerve activity in the brain. Rigor mortis sets in quite quickly after death (but do not confuse it with certain rigid conditions during fits etc.) and it tends to disappear again after perhaps twenty-four hours. Do not take responsibility for judging whether or not an animal is dead: get expert diagnosis, and in the meantime do all you can to sustain life. It is always better to treat a dead body than to fail to treat a living one.

If the animal is **conscious,** it is bound to be fearful and in danger of causing itself further injury or later collapse if it panics. It might also damage you, either by direct self-defensive attack or by flailing its wings or limbs or unwittingly swinging its horns or antlers. Be firm, kind and calm so that you are psychologically in control and can gain the animal's confidence and acquiescence, but also be prepared to secure it physically if necessary for its own good.

RESUSCITATION

Check whether or not the animal is breathing; make sure that it is possible for it to breathe and to continue to do so. Check that the nostrils are cleared and that there are no obstructions in the throat or mouth. Breathing might be obstructed by the presence of foreign objects such as a piece of food or bone, a half-swallowed fragment of broken tooth, or some fishing tackle; or by the animal's own vomit, water in the lungs during drowning, a noose of some kind (snare, tight collar, fishing line), a swollen sting in the mouth or throat, a broken neck, pressure on the windpipe, the action of certain poisons like strychnine or carbon monoxide, or the collapse of the animal's lungs from injury, shock or pneumonia.

An unconscious animal will need help to maintain or restart its breathing. Once you have cleared any obstructions from the airways, draw its tongue forward and align its head for a clear air passage. There may be blood or mucus in the throat, which needs to be carefully swabbed out with damp, compressed cottonwool or, in the case of a small creature, sucked out by means of a straw or tube. Act fast: life is at risk.

If an animal has been rescued from **drowning,** the immediate need is to drain the water from its lungs. A smaller animal can be held upside down by its hind legs to drain the lungs and, if necessary, it can be swung from side to side or even in circles so that centrifugal force gives added effect. A larger animal should be placed on its side on a slope so that the hindquarters are uphill from its head, then you should kneel on the upper part of its chest (you will need to put your whole weight on something like a horse or cow) so that the fluid drains from its mouth. When no more is flowing, turn the animal on to its other side and repeat the procedure.

Resuscitation techniques include intermittent pressure on the rib cage (unless it is broken, badly damaged or vulnerable), mouth-to-mouth blowing, and indirect methods like rocking the body or, in the case of new-born mammals, the use of slight pain to encourage the animal to gasp and draw its first breath (pinch an ear, perhaps, or slap its chest if it is the size of a calf).

In the case of an unconscious casualty which has stopped breathing, the aim of artificial respiration is to remove carbon dioxide from its lungs and allow them to fill with oxygen instead. This is usually done by **pressing on the chest** at intervals—perhaps ten to twenty times in a minute, depending on how big the animal is and at what rate it would normally take its breaths. If an animal is deprived of oxygen, it very quickly succumbs to brain damage and heart failure, so you must act fast.

Lie the animal on its right sight and kneel beside it. Spread your hands over its ribs, just behind the shoulder blade, and keep your arms straight as you rock some of your weight forwards to apply firm pressure over the rib cage, then promptly rock back to allow the lungs to fill with air. Keep your feet in contact with the ground even if it is a large animal such as a cow or horse. Rock forward again at intervals—perhaps five or six seconds after the release in the case of a dog. The release part of the action is just as important as the pressing: the latter empties the lungs of carbon dioxide and the former allows them to fill naturally with oxygen.

This method can be used with animals the size of a fox or larger. For smaller animals, including cats, only one hand is needed to press and release the rib cage at intervals. But even this will be too heavy-handed for those that have delicate rib cages. A bird, for example, should be put on a flat surface and its body rocked so that its head rises and falls, which will encourage the air sacs to function. Or put a wedge (perhaps a horizontal piece of wood, making sure that it cannot be inadvertently swallowed) to keep the bird's beak ajar, lay it carefully on a stable surface, belly down, with its neck gently extended to open the air passages, put your hand lightly over its back so that your thumb is on one side of its thorax (chest) and your fingers on the other, and then exert gentle pressure on the thorax by squeezing lightly every fifteen to twenty seconds and releasing. Take great care with a bird: the bone structure is necessarily light, and apart from damaging the rib cage itself there is also the risk of internal injury to vital organs.

For **mouth-to-mouth resuscitation** of a small animal, cup your hand to channel your breath and blow direct into the animal's mouth. Use only enough to expand the chest to its normal size. Do not use mouth-to-mouth if you suspect the animal is diseased or has been poisoned or gassed.

Once breathing has started, keep the animal warm and very quiet, and monitor its progress continually so that resuscitation can be given again if it is needed.

Table I gives the normal rate of respiration for several species. Broadly speaking, the larger the animal, the fewer breaths it takes in a given period. However, many factors affect the rate of breathing, especially in a distressed animal. During unconsciousness, breathing tends to be slower, whereas a conscious animal in a state of shock has shallow, fast breathing. If it is suffering from hypothermia (severe cooling of the body) its breathing will be shallow but slow. Young animals normally breathe faster than adults, and females tend to breathe faster than males, especially when pregnant.

CARDIAC ARREST

Cardiac arrest, or heart failure, tends to occur some time after breathing has stopped—perhaps ten minutes later in the case of, say, a chicken. If the heart has stopped beating completely—and only if you can quite literally detect not even the faintest hint of a beat or pulse—you could try external **heart massage.** With big animals, this requires vigorous action and is not for the timid.

TABLE I
NORMAL TEMPERATURES, RESPIRATION AND PULSE RATES

	Normal Temperature (average °C)	Respiration Rate (per minute)	Pulse Rate (per minute)
Birds			
Fowl size	41.6	35 – 40	Too high for
Small birds	42.5	100 – 150 +	accurate measurement
Mammals			
Cat	38.4	20 – 30	110 – 120
Cattle	38.9	12 – 16	45 – 50
Dog	38.3	15 – 30	90 – 100
Ferret	38.8		
Gerbil	38.0		
Guinea pig	38.6		
Goat	40.0	12 – 20	70 – 80
Hamster	37.5		
Horse	38.0	8 – 12	32 – 42
Mouse	37.5		130 – 150
Pig	39.7	10 – 16	70 – 80
Rabbit	38.4		
Rat	38.0		
Sheep	40.0	12 – 20	70 – 80

The aim is to apply sudden pressure over the heart area at intervals similar to those of the animal's natural pulse rate when in good health. Pulse rate (or rates of heart beat) are shown in Table I.

Heart massage is not easy unless you have experience, and you must be absolutely certain that the heart has in fact stopped beating completely before you try it. You might need to practise artificial respiration at the same time, which complicates matters. However, to give heart massage to animals like a fox, dog, cat, badger, sheep and pig, put both hands (one on top of the other) over the animal's breastbone or sternum, press firmly and quite sharply downwards and forwards over the heart, maintain that pressure for about a second, then release. Repeat the action after a couple of seconds, and continue with this rhythm but stop the moment you detect a pulse. For a bird as big as a swan or eagle, place it on its back and put your palms on either side of the heart area, then press them simultaneously; retain the pressure for a second, then relax for a second and repeat. For an animal as big as a horse or cow, you could in desperation try a solid thump with both your knees over the heart area.

Heart attacks in any animal are the result of a reduction in the supply of blood to the heart. The animal will be in a state of shock and possible collapse; its pulse will be weak and irregular, its breath will probably be short, and you are likely to see a blue tinge (termed cyanosis) to membranes—check lips, gums and tongue for colour. Lay the animal down, clear its airways and apply artificial respiration if necessary, or cardiac massage if the heart has stopped. In the meantime make sure that the vet has been summoned as a matter of urgency.

UNCONSCIOUSNESS

There are varying degrees of unconsciousness, which can arise from a wide range of situations including concussion, fits of various kinds, shock, certain types of poisoning, hysteria, hypothermia, heat stroke, electrocution, suffocation, drowning, heart attack or severe brain injury.

Concussion, or stunning, is a temporary condition, typically caused by a blow to the head in an RTA or by a bird flying into a window-pane. The animal is dazed and confused, if not actually unconscious, but its eyes do react to the stimulus of light or touch, though the pupils will probably be small. It might suffer temporarily from blindness.

If the only problem is stunning, the animal will recover of its own accord in due course, perhaps in minutes or perhaps an hour or two. Put it somewhere warm and dark, with as much peace and privacy as possible. It will of course need protection from predators until it has regained its senses fully. As it "comes round", it will be as groggy as a boxer but should in fact suffer no permanent after effects.

A more severe injury to the skull or brain could lead to a longer, **deeper unconsciousness** and the animal will not only be confused when it finally comes round but will probably suffer loss of balance and could also be blind. If there is brain haemorrhage, there might also be paralysis. Give the animal a quiet environment, preferably in subdued light, and keep an eye on its breathing and pulse, being prepared to give artificial respiration or cardiac massage as soon as it is needed.

In a more profound **coma,** the unconsciousness is deep and there will be no reflexes at all to external stimuli. This is typical of some diabetes patients, and can also arise from very high temperatures, poisoning and of course brain injury.

If an unconscious animal is rigid rather than relaxed, it might be suffering from some kind of a **fit.** This category includes epilepsy and the type of fits associated with pregnancy or lactation (milk fever). Fits can also be caused by something as apparently mundane as internal parasites or teething. Lead poisoning is another possible cause of fits.

An animal in the throes of muscular spasm during a fit should not be handled or restrained but do make sure it cannot injure itself during the convulsions, for example on something hot or sharp. Keep the environment dark and very quiet; try and surround the animal with cushioning to prevent limb damage; and above all make sure it is not subjected to any sudden noises, which could be fatal to it. Leave it alone in a dark room to recover, and ask for veterinary advice.

WOUNDS AND BLEEDING

An injured animal might bleed obviously from external wounds or, more dangerously, internally from damage to various organs such as the liver or spleen or the rupture of a large blood vessel. Symptoms of **internal bleeding** include *very* pale mouth and mucous membranes (for example, eyelids), cold skin, rapid breathing and possibly a series of gasps, general listlessness and apathy. The pulse becomes so weak and slow that it is eventually imperceptible and the animal will collapse. If the bleeding is severe, it will prove almost impossible to save the animal's life: its temperature drops, it begins to twitch, its eyes become glazed, convulsions begin and these lead to coma and death. If the animal vomits a considerable quantity of blood, it has a very serious stomach injury or disease and you are unlikely to save it. Any bleeding from the mouth or nose could indicate problems, and any degree of internal bleeding needs urgent veterinary treatment; while you wait for the vet, keep the animal warm, calm, very quiet and reassured.

Reassurance is also needed for animals with **external wounds.** Check the coat or plumage for matted blood on hair or feathers in case the wound is not immediately obvious. There are several types of wound:

- Incisions:
  Clean cuts by a sharp instrument such as a knife or a piece of glass or metal. Bleeding is profuse but is easily controlled and soon stops.
- Punctures:
  Caused by a pointed instrument such as spikes, nails, canine or incisor teeth during an attack or fight, also entry of bullet or pellet. Needs veterinary attention—easily becomes infected and can be deceptively deep, however small the external wound.

- Lacerations:
  Jagged, torn areas of flesh (typical of barbed-wire wounds). Usually very painful for a few days, often suppurates, and leaves scars. Needs veterinary attention and should not be disturbed if the blood has already clotted over the wound.
- Abrasions:
  Grazing—loss of outer skin layers (think of small boys' knees!).
- Contusions:
  Bruising, for example from kicks, blows from a stick, RTAs. Not much sign of external bleeding: the bleeding is under the skin and there is much bruising of surrounding tissues. Responds to cold compress.
- Closed wounds:
  Entry hole has sealed foreign body within the wound—typically bullets, thorns, pellets, glass, fish hooks. Definitely one for the vet.

The actual bleeding (or haemorrhage) of a wound can be classified by the colour and flow pattern of the blood:

- Arterial:
  Bright scarlet, spurting out in time with the heartbeat. Arterial bleeding can sometimes stop of its own accord because of a fall in blood pressure due to shock.
- Venous:
  Dark in colour, and flowing: the blood wells up from the depths of a wound in a steady stream.
- Capillary:
  Oozes gradually from a slight injury and soon stops of its own accord because of clotting.

To stop bleeding, apply pressure. In the case of a large vessel, pressure should be applied from above the wound if the source is an artery but below if it is a vein. (Remember: arteries spurt, veins flow.) Use your finger in an emergency until you can apply a pressure pad of some kind over the wound—perhaps a clean piece of sheet or a pillowcase for a large animal, or a handerkerchief for a small one. Press the pad over the wound, and maintain the pressure for about a quarter of an hour. With a big wound, you might be able to press a clean finger and thumb where the blood is issuing if that point is visible, then use a moist, clean pressure pad pressed into the wound with your hand or by firm bandaging. Birds, by the way, can only afford to lose a few *drops* of blood, but their blood does tend to clot quickly: apply a pressure pad (something like surgical gauze) or help clotting of seeping bleeding by using a styptic.

Tourniquets should only be applied if other methods of arresting the bleeding fail, and in any event they should *never* be left on for more than twenty minutes or the limb will be permanently damaged. Only use a tourniquet in an emergency if you know what you are doing and if the haemorrhage is serious. For most animals you can make a tourniquet from a rolled handkerchief: knot it round the limb and tighten it by slipping a pencil under it and twisting it tight—just tight enough to stop the bleeding, but no tighter than that. For larger livestock you could use a length of *soft* rope or rubber tubing. Tourniquets should be released *slowly*.

It helps if you cut away hair around a wound to avoid subsequent matting and possible suppuration. **To clean the surface of a wound,** use a warm solution of salt and water (or possibly a warm dilution of TCP, Savlon or Centrimide if the wound is not to be sutured). Leave the wound clean and unbandaged if it is to be seen by the vet, but it might be necessary to apply a dry dressing to protect it from flies and dirt. Do not try and remove a projecting foreign object: you will probably make matters worse. Seek veterinary help instead.

Minor wounds like scratches and grazes are often best treated by the animal's own saliva as it licks them, or you can bathe them with plain warm water to remove all traces of dirt, then bathe gently in a saline solution of a teaspoonful of salt in a pint of water.

If a wound is hot, painful or discoloured, it is already infected—whether or not pus is present. If it stinks, it is probably gangrenous and it certainly needs veterinary treatment.

Watch out for **shot wounds,** which can look deceptively minor on the outside. Shotgun wounds result in a spread of several pellets and are mostly near the surface if a gun is fired from a distance. Airgun slugs are single pellets and leave only a small hole but can shatter bone even so. The bullet from, say, a .22 will also leave a small entry hole but can pass right through the body, leaving a typically large and messy exit hole. The bolt of a crossbow is pretty unmistakable and often lethal, but many victims are found alive with the bolt sticking right through their necks or bodies.

Embedded **barbed fish hooks** cannot and should not be pulled back out again the way they entered because the barbs will cause considerable damage by ripping into the surrounding area. A hook through the webbing of a bird's foot (or of your own hand) is best removed by gently pushing it further through in the same direction as the point of the hook until you can cut off the barbed end, then you can withdraw the thing quite easily. If it is embedded in the soft part of the beak, a hook can often be removed with the careful use of pliers if the incision is a recent one, but if it is already infected or if the hook is deeper into the beak or down into the throat or gizzard, the bird must have veterinary attention for its removal.

Amphibians and reptiles often manage to survive quite severe wounding and many a vet has experience of stitching up exotic species kept as pets or amputating when necessary; they can apply this experience to wild native species. Animals like lizards are happy enough to part with their tails as an escape mechanism in the teeth of a predator and no treatment is necessary: somehow the tail will probably grow again. Many insects are also capable of regenerating lost extremities. With birds and mammals, of course, the situation is much more serious and you need to consider the implications of severe limb damage, especially for wild creatures. Amputation is certainly possible, but it might be kinder in the long run to have the victim put down instead, especially those for which anaesthesia might be dangerous.

SHOCK

Any distressed animal is likely to be in a state of shock to a greater or lesser degree, and as already mentioned it is often the effects of shock upon close contact with a human rescuer that kills a wild creature rather than its original injuries. Some domestic species are just as vulnerable.

Shock is characterised by an abrupt fall in blood pressure, and its symptoms include a drop in body temperature, betrayed by cold extremities but without any shivering (this is sometimes preceded by an initial rise in temperature, and a mammal will pant and have a hot, dry nose), a fast but weak pulse and rapid, shallow breathing. Membranes such as lips, tongue, gums and eye sockets are usually very pale, but this can also indicate internal bleeding which means that any attempt to move the animal could be fatal to it. If the membranes have a blue tinge, there could be a shortage of oxygen in the blood, but this "cyanosis" colouring can also be the result of nitrite poisoning, and is typical in the case of asphyxia from smoke and fumes.

Other possible symptoms of shock are vomiting and uncontrolled urination and bowel movements, hysteria, great thirst, general weakness or even unconsciousness, but it is body temperature, breathing, pulse and pallor that are the more reliable guides to the animal's problem. A bird is typically weak, listless, and cold to the touch; it will have pale membranes and a slow pulse and you should be aware that the shock reaction is often delayed in a bird, sometimes by as much as a couple of days.

Do not move a shocked animal unless it is essential to do so. The most important first aid is to keep it in a warm, dark, quiet, comfortable environment: it needs privacy, security and the opportunity to rest, preferably in subdued light. Make sure its airways are unrestricted and are kept clear of vomit. Wild species should be given complete isolation to avoid additional upset; domesticated animals will also appreciate privacy and need adequate reassurance and calmness from a familiar handler.

The proper diagnosis, understanding and treatment of shock are vital to a distressed animal's eventual recovery and, after the immediate saving of life, treatment of shock should be your priority. In many cases the animal will be dehydrated: if it is conscious and thirsty, gently encourage it to drink glucose in water or a rehydration fluid like Lectade, but do not pressurise it to do so, and *never* force liquids into an unconscious animal: you will drown it.

FRACTURES

Fractures fall into two break categories: either *simple,* in which there is a clean break right across the bone, with no damage to the skin; or *compound,* in which the skin is injured, often by the bone protruding through, and which can result in infection and severe bleeding.

The obvious symptoms of fractures include an inability to use the affected part, an unnatural appearance in mobility, obvious deformity, swelling, and pain on moving. A vet will probably check for crepitus of fragments—which is as unpleasant as it sounds (the grating noise of bone pieces against each other) and should not be tried by amateurs.

Always be very careful if you have to move an animal with any kind of fracture: you must avoid jarring it in any way, both because of the pain this can cause and because it could complicate the injury. Ideally, in the case of an animal with a broken leg, carry the patient in such a way that its limbs dangle down naturally under its body, with its back uppermost, so that the force of gravity takes the pressure off the fractured bone. For example, carry a dog or calf by putting one arm around the back of its buttocks and the other around the front of its chest to support the body weight, leaving the legs trailing down. If you must lay the animal down or need to use a stretcher so that it is lying on its side, avoid letting the broken limb dangle sideways from the body (which is an unnatural alignment) and therefore make sure that it is supported from underneath at all stages, either by the other limb or by the surface on which the animal is lying.

If the broken bone is protruding through the flesh, carefully but quite firmly and steadily stretch the limb in the natural direction so that the bone can slip back out of sight, or at least cushion the limb during transport (but without letting the padding touch the exposed bone) in order to protect it from jarring and from any accidental contact which would complicate the injury by introducing infection into the bone matter.

If any part of the spine is fractured the slightest movement could result in fatality. In any case, spinal injuries cause such intense pain that an animal which is not already completely paralysed will be uncharacteristically and violently aggressive towards you. If it proves essential to move an animal with spinal damage, carry it with extreme care and consideration on a *firm* blanket stretcher. If you suspect such an injury it is much better to wait for veterinary diagnosis and help.

For any animal with a suspected fracture, reassurance is the most important first-aid treatment and it also helps if you can keep the patient warm. Simple limb fractures seem to cause less distress to animals than to human patients: they do not seem to have our psychological problems with pain and many wild animals experience complete and successful healing of fractured bones in the wild without any help at all.

However, in general the quicker a fracture can be accurately diagnosed and professionally treated, the more likely it is to heal successfully, especially if such treatment can be applied before there is any swelling. On no account should you try and splint a fractured bone yourself unless you are experienced: you will cause more pain than relief and will probably make the fracture worse.

Amphibians' broken bones will heal of their own accord, but slowly, and it helps if the animal has access to water so that the weight is taken off the fracture. Reptiles, especially lizards, seem quite often to suffer from fractures and veterinary advice should be sought. Chelonians (tortoises, turtles etc.) can fracture their shells, which can generally be repaired with an epoxy resin. Oh that bones were so simple!

DISLOCATIONS

The symptoms of dislocated joints are in many ways similar to those of fractures: there may be loss of or reduction in function of the joint, pain if it is moved, and swelling around it. There may also be obvious deformity. Veterinary treatment is necessary but in the meantime make the animal comfortable in a confined space to deter movement. You can apply cold compresses to soothe the joint but it is better not to bandage it.

BURNS AND SCALDS

Animals can suffer burns from dry heat sources like fire, lightning and electricity, from corrosive acids and alkalis, friction (like rope burns), or wet sources which cause scalding. Typical evidence of burns includes singed hair or feathers as well as great pain, whereas scalds might show little superficial evidence of their presence for several hours or even a couple of days, and might also be hidden by a scab.

The immediate concern with burns and scalds is to reduce the heat of the affected body tissues by plunging the area into cold water and keeping it immersed for ten or fifteen minutes. Once the flesh has cooled, it can be covered with a dry, clean bandage or cloth but do not use any kind of oil or lotion to try and soothe it, though you could usefully soak the cloth in very strong tea. This contains tannic acids which encourage the rapid formation of a protective coagulum over the wound. Even better, keep a tube of tannic acid jelly in your first-aid kit, but only use it for small burns. Very large areas can be covered with clean cloths soaked in a mild saline solution.

Bear in mind that, once it has been burned, the damaged tissue is very vulnerable to infection—you should not even breathe on it—and will have very little resistance to bacterial attack; it is also likely to induce toxaemia (blood poisoning). However, the biggest problem is likely to be shock and the animal needs to be given a calm, isolated, warm environment in which to recover, with ample reassurance if it is a domesticated pet. Offer it water to drink but do not force it to do so. Good nursing, both at this stage and during convalescence, is the secret of successful treatment in burn cases.

Veterinary assistance should be requested as a matter of urgency so that the animal's pain can be reduced, the effects of shock counteracted and the wound itself professionally treated. There are five recognised degrees of burns, and really only the first (mildest) degree might not need veterinary treatment.

If the burns are caused by corrosive acids or alkalis, you need to neutralise the substance as well as remove it with all possible speed—certainly before the animal can lick or preen itself and end up with burnt membranes in the mouth and throat which could swell up and cause asphyxia, and certainly before the stuff poisons it. Flood the mouth as well as the coat, paws etc., with cold water to dilute and flush away the contaminant. Details of antidotes and neutralisers are given in the 'Poisons' section below, but the basic principle is that an acid substance will neutralise an alkaline one, and vice versa. Use the neutraliser with copious amounts of water to sluice the corrosive substance off the skin. Use milk or bicarbonate of soda (2 parts bicarbonate to 98 of water) to neutralise acids; use weak vinegar (5 parts to 95 of water) to neutralise alkalis like caustic soda and ammonia.

ELECTROCUTION

Typical situations involving electrocution are birds flying into high tension cables, lightning strikes, and accidents with mains electricity. If the animal is still in contact with a live supply of electricity, *switch off the current* before you touch the animal or you, too, will be electrocuted. If you cannot locate the source of supply, use a *wooden* walking-stick to pull the animal clear of contact.

The major problem with **electrocution** (assuming the animal lives) is shock and in some cases resuscitation will be needed if breathing has ceased or the heart has stopped. Keep the animal warm and peaceful; give fluids if it can accept them (but be careful of causing additional stress to a wild animal). There might also be burns to be treated, and perhaps fractures. Always seek urgent veterinary help with electrocution cases.

With **lightning strikes,** the most likely result is instant death and quite often cattle in particular are found dead in the field, sometimes near the tree under which they had taken shelter from the storm, but frequently out in the open. Singe marks might be apparent, or there might be no clue at all to the deaths. In the rare cases where cattle survive lightning strikes, they will appear to be partially or wholly paralysed, as though there was spinal injury, and will be very agitated. There might be singe marks, especially on the back and shoulders and sometimes on the legs, and the skin near these marks will be deeply and extensively bruised.

HEATSTROKE

This is a situation in which an animal, usually of a domesticated species, is unable to reduce its own body temperature adequately. Typical problems, nearly always caused by human neglect, are dogs shut in cars with the sun beating down, ferrets in similar situations, or pets from temperate regions suddenly finding themselves in tropical climates after the stress of a long journey and the bewilderment of alien surroundings. Certain deer confined to a building and rushing about in a panic will also succumb to overheating.

The signs are obvious distress, excessive panting, and a sudden and great lethargy which might induce the animal to stagger about and to fall over if forced to move. Its body temperature will be extremely high and there may be loss of consciousness or convulsions.

Very fast action must be taken to save the animal's life as heatstroke is a killer and death is possible within a few hours although it may take up to three days. First of all remove the animal from the overheated environment to a cool place and then do everything possible to reduce its body heat fast: use a hose to douche with cold water, and apply frequently-changed, soaking wet cold pads or sheets; get paws into cold water; use ice-cubes with smaller animals; and try to create cold air for the animal to breathe (the quickest way to cool the body is via the lungs). Keep applying the cooling treatment until an unconscious animal comes round and make sure it can breathe: pull its tongue forward.

In the meantime someone should be summoning the vet as a matter of urgency. If the animal does recover, it is likely to remain weak and dull for several weeks.

HYPOTHERMIA

Hypothermia is the opposite extreme to heatstroke: it is a severe cooling of the body temperature. The most vulnerable are the very small, the new-born and the very old, and the most likely circumstances leading to hypothermia are prolonged exposure to the cold, particularly a long period in cold or icy water. It can also be the result of certain types of poisoning or drugs. The animal's body temperature will be very low; its pulse will be so weak and slow that you can hardly feel it, and its breathing will be slow and shallow. It is in a state of collapse and you must act immediately, while you are waiting urgently for the vet. Warm it up: get it into a warm environment, cover it with blankets, massage its body to help circulation; and stand by to give artificial respiration if its breathing is interrupted, or cardiac massage if the heart stops beating completely.

FROST-BITE

Exposure to severe cold for long periods causes the body to restrict its superficial blood vessels so that it can maintain body temperature and minimise heat loss. Extremities such as ear tips and tails (or poultry wattles and combs) are thus made susceptible to freezing and become completely numb. A bird's feet, for example, will become red and swollen. Sometimes you would not suspect frost-bite until in due course the affected areas become gangrenous and drop off.

The frost-bitten area will not be painful while it remains numb but will hurt as the part thaws out. Warm the animal very gradually: do not plunge the damaged area into hot water or rub it with snow.   '

POISONS

The causes and symptoms of poisoning are so varied that the problem needs rapid expert attention. It is important that the poisonous substance be identified accurately and you must therefore get proper veterinary diagnosis and treatment.

Gases

Typically dangerous emissions in enclosed spaces are car exhaust fumes and the fumes from gas or solid-fuel boilers and heaters where ventilation is inadequate—in both cases the gas is carbon monoxide, which is sometimes used anyway for the destruction of certain animals. Other lethal and quick-killing substances are the fumes released by certain kinds of furniture foam when burning, or acrolein fumes from overheating cooking fats in a confined space. There have also been cases of cage birds and domestic pets dying from fumes given off by dry non-stick pans left unattended on the stove, and there are several gases used to exterminate "vermin" like rats and moles.

If an animal is subjected to poisonous fumes, your first and vital step is to get it away from the poisoned environment and out into really fresh air. Then check that its air passages are free. With luck, fresh air will itself effect the cure and you only need to give treatment for shock, but if the animal is unconscious or in a state of collapse you should summon veterinary help immediately and give resuscitation in the meantime. Do *not* use mouth-to-mouth resuscitation: you will probably draw the poisonous gases into your own lungs.

Ingested Poisons

The aim when dealing with ingested poisons is to reduce their absorption into body tissues as fast as you can. With some substances this will be by giving **emetics** to cause vomiting or purgatives to stimulate the bowels, but in many cases such violent measures will cause more harm than good and your aim will be to neutralise the poison appropriately. Veterinary measures might include stomach pumping, injections and fluid therapy. Do not try and make an animal vomit if corrosive acids have been ingested and have therefore inflamed its mouth and throat. In these and many other cases you will need to give a demulcent (to soothe the membranes) once the poison has been diluted or neutralised.

Where appropriate, emetics likely to be found around the house include salt with water (about two tablespoonsful to the cup), washing soda (a lump the size of a hazel nut for a dog or cat), Epsom salts, or mustard in water (about a dessertspoonful in a cupful of water for a pig).

Demulcents include milk, raw eggs, olive oil and liquid paraffin. In many cases the animal will also benefit from the tannic acid in strong black tea or coffee which has been boiled: the tannins counteract the effect of vegetable poisons by hindering their absorption in livestock like cattle, sheep and horses. They can also be used as stimulants to counteract the effect of narcotic poisoning from, say, barbiturates, and have a role to play in emergency first aid for poisoning by those two potential killers, strychnine and lead.

Some of the first-aid steps in the case of certain more common poisons are given below, but do bear in mind that, unless you actually *know* that the animal has ingested a poison and what that poison is, only a veterinary surgeon can be sure that symptoms are in fact indicative of poisoning (many could be of various other problems). In nearly every case of poisoning, whatever the substance, veterinary treatment is likely to be more effective more quickly than anything you can do yourself.

Acids   Act at once. Do not use emetics or try any other means of making the animal vomit. Act fast to neutralise the acid by giving alkaline demulcents like bicarbonate of soda or chalk, in barleywater or milk: these will also soothe the animal's membranes. If you have nothing else, give plenty of water to try and dilute the acid and minimise its corrosiveness. If the animal is unconscious, do not force liquid down the throat as it is bound to enter the windpipe and drown the patient. Many acids have specific antidotes.

Alkalis   Less likely problem than acids, but include substances like ammonia, caustic soda and potash. Neutralise with very dilute acids like weak vinegar.

Alphachloralose   Typical bait for woodpigeons and mice, with hypnotic and stupefying effects. You must use emetics within half an hour of ingestion. The animal is susceptible to hypothermia and must be kept warm.

Arsenic   Irritant leading to gastro-enteritis: can be very rapid in effect and you must get the vet immediately. Your only first-aid hope is to induce vomiting (in species which can vomit) with a strong solution of salt and water. Veterinary treatment includes specific antidotes, usually given intravenously.

Barbiturates   If not unconscious, give emetics (or stomach pump) and artificial respiration; keep warm; give strong coffee.

Lead   A major problem for cattle (who seem to love the taste of lead paint) and wildfowl (not just anglers' lead weights but also shotgun pellets picked up as gizzard grit while grazing). Lead is as lethal in very old, flaking paint as in discarded paint-tins, and is also found in tarpaulins and in the form of red lead used by some plumbers. Symptoms of lead poisoning can be dramatic and alarming, and often include paralysis. Two pieces of ingested lead shot can kill a pigeon; ten can kill a swan slowly, or a goose. Pigs, on the other hand, can eat a dose of lead which would kill a cow without showing any effects at all.

First-aid treatment for mammals (not birds) includes large doses of Epsom salts (magnesium sulphate), milk, egg whites or strong tea. Keep the animal warm and quiet while you wait for veterinary treatment with specific antidotes.

Metaldehyde   Often used in slug pellets, and often picked up by dogs, cats, birds, sheep, cattle and horses. Veterinary treatment is essential. Keep the animal quiet and in the dark, and if it is already experiencing muscular spasm it is *essential* that it is not subjected to sudden noises, which will kill it.

Pesticides and Herbicides   There are so many different substances used for killing insects, weeds and just about every other living thing you can think of that it is difficult to give specific advice should such substances be ingested by an animal. Get veterinary help immediately, especially in the case of something like Paraquat, but in the meantime try and keep the animal still to avoid increasing its body's absorption of the poison, and keep it warm. Do not use an emetic but you could try diluting with drinks of milk and water. An unexpected source of pesticides might be fruit-tree sprays drifting from orchards or being ingested by livestock which graze orchards. Another source is the inappropriate use of some flea powders, especially on young puppies and kittens, or carelessly on hedgehogs. If you think you know what has caused the poisoning, take the container's label to the vet for information about the contents.

Phenol   Includes carbolic acid, coal tar antiseptics, creosote, Lysol, pitch etc. For treatment of skin, see section on 'Pollution' in Chapter 4 (phenols can be all too easily absorbed through the skin and must be removed quickly, especially in the case of cats). The substances are often ingested during a contaminated animal's attempts to clean itself and they are corrosive, leading to shock, convulsions and death. Give oral demulcents like milk or raw egg white.

Phosphorus   This might be ingested from, say, rat poison or chewed matches. You must act very quickly indeed: death can be within hours. Any vomit is often green and appears to be luminous in the dark. The animal will have acute pain in its abdomen and an intense thirst (it will also have diarrhoea) but will be very lethargic. Give an immediate emetic—but do *not* use any fats, oils, egg whites or milk, all of which enable the poison to be absorbed more readily by the animal's body. Use bluestone (copper sulphate) to induce vomiting, and repeat the dose every fifteen minutes.

Poisonous Plants   There are many plants which are poisonous, especially to herbivorous livestock, and the symptoms and treatments vary according to what has been eaten. Another source of food poisoning is feeding one species with medicated foods designed for another. The infamous yew plant has a highly poisonous seed in its berry but the flesh of the berry itself is harmless, and delicious.

Strychnine   The symptoms of strychnine poisoning are usually violent— alarming convulsions with the animal arching its spine backwards so that its head is pulled back.

Act very fast indeed. Summon the vet as a matter of extreme urgency and in the meantime give the animal an absolutely quiet environment: the slightest noise or stimulus could be fatal. The vet will probably anaesthetise the animal and either pump its stomach or inject an emetic; you could try very strong tea in the meantime for a large animal, or a suitable emetic for a smaller one as soon as you notice the problem.

Warfarin   This anti-coagulant rodenticide causes internal bleeding in rats and mice, and occasional cases of accidental poisoning of domestic animals have also been reported. There is also the problem that, as with strychnine, the substance can linger in urine, which might then further contaminate food. If you know an animal has ingested Warfarin, there is absolutely nothing you can do yourself and you must get veterinary assistance: the treatment involves injections of vitamin K1 and probably a blood transfusion. In the meantime be very gentle in your handling of the animal, because otherwise you might aggravate the internal bleeding.

Injected Poisons

In the case of **bee and wasp stings,** veterinary treatment will be needed if the sting is in the throat or mouth, which might swell up and restrict breathing, or in the eye, ear or anus. In other cases, remove the sting carefully (bees leave their stings in their victims) and use one of the following remedies: apply a drop or two of ammonia, or a creamy paste of bicarbonate of soda; rub with half a freshly cut onion; hold a blue-bag against it; or simply soothe the area with a cold-water compress.

The only poisonous snake native to Britain is the adder, though there is always the slight risk of coming across an escaped exotic species. **Bites from adders** are comparatively rare as the snake would much prefer to escape than attack, but dogs do sometimes get bitten, especially sporting dogs intent on their work, and might die; so in some cases might livestock—sheep, cattle and horses, but not pigs—though more often the animal suffers an uncomfortably swollen leg rather than fatality.

The symptoms of an adder bite include considerable swelling, local pain, livid colouring around the bite, and lameness if a limb has been bitten. The victim will probably be rather frightened and should be reassured and kept calm; get veterinary assistance immediately. Try using a tourniquet to prevent the poison spreading—but only for a short while (see 'Wounds' above).

Poisoned Birds

John Cooper, in his classic book *First Aid and Care of Wild Birds,* advises that it is essential to remove any poisons from the crop or stomach of a bird by sucking the stuff out or washing it out with the aid of a stomach tube and a little warm water (ask a vet to show you how). A useful antidote, given by stomach tube to absorb the poison and neutralise its direct effects, would be a mixture of 10 g activated charcoal, 5 g kaolin, 5 g light magnesium oxide and 5 g tannic acid, combined with water to make 500 ml of solution and then given orally at the rate of 2-20 ml, depending on the size of the bird. He also suggests the use of very strong cold tea to precipitate many metallic and alkaloid poisons; tincture of iodine for some metals; lime water to neutralise acids; dilute vinegar for alkalis; and a diluted solution of the purple disinfectant, potassium permanganate, to deal with phosphorus compounds. Cooper's book is a bible which should be on the shelf of every wild-bird hospital or sanctuary in the land.

EYES, EARS AND NOSES

Saline washes (a teaspoonful of salt in a pint of lukewarm water) are useful for eye problems. To remove a foreign body from an animal's eye requires considerable delicacy and an amenable patient. Put a little eye ointment on the tip of your finger so that the mote adheres to it and you can lift it out. If you see a hedgehog running around in circles with its eyes tightly shut, they might be full of maggots. Bathe the eyes with warm water to ungum the lids, then take a look to check the damage. Any maggots should be plucked out with a pair of blunt forceps.

Foreign bodies in ears are indicated when an animal shakes and rubs it head, or holds its head to one side. Unless you are experienced, do not try and remove the obstruction yourself but ask for veterinary assistance. In an emergency you could dribble a little warm olive oil into the ear. A more common ear problem (parasites apart) is superficial bleeding as a result of fights or arguments with brambles, and sometimes the bleeding is quite profuse. Try a cold compress to reduce it.

Nose bleeds might be the result of a blow or of illness. A cold compress held against the muzzle for a quarter of an hour could help, but you must be aware that such bleeding could indicate serious trouble and will need proper diagnosis.

NURSING

Good nursing has saved many an animal which a vet might have advised should be put down. The essentials are a realistic empathy with the patient, an understanding of its behaviour and needs, an appropriate environment, peace and privacy, scrupulous attention to hygiene, careful feeding, and the ability to know almost instinctively when something is not quite right. A major problem in nursing wildlife is to avoid "humanising" an animal that will be returned to the wild when it is fit; another problem is that many animals will only trust one person, so that your duties becomes full-time.

Do make use of vets and listen to their advice, even if you eventually decide not to follow it to the letter. However, most veterinary drugs have only been tested for use on domesticated species, or perhaps zoo animals, and in many cases very little is known about their use for wildlife. Several wildlife hospitals have found **homoeopathy** more acceptable and successful: at worst it does no harm, and it often seems to give quicker results in certain situations. Homoeopathy is an art rather than a science and it is difficult to lay down hard and fast rules about dosages. If you do use homoeopathy, keep careful records and make sure your data is published to help others—your failures as well as your successes.

Medications, homoeopathic or otherwise, can be given by mouth or by injection. The inexperienced should give **injections** only under veterinary instruction and supervision, until they are both competent and confident. To give **pills, pellets and powders** orally, the first idea might be to disguise the medication in some tempting food but this fools very few animals and they are likely to refuse to eat the "contaminated" food, or to spit it out. Cats and dogs are notoriously clever at pretending to swallow a pill, keeping it carefully in their mouths until they can discreetly get rid of it.

To make sure that a dose is swallowed properly, open the patient's mouth or beak and put the medication right at the back of the throat. Wrap it up in a pellet of food if you like, or perhaps oil it a little to help it slide down the gullet. Then close the mouth and, keeping it firmly closed, encourage the animal to swallow by stroking its throat until you are certain it has gone the way it should. (See Fig. 40 on p. 136 for oral dosing for a cat.)

Liquids, or powders or crushed pills dissolved in liquids, can be easier to give than pills and will not be spat out. Force-feed the liquid by inserting the end of a non-chewable dosing tube, syringe or dropper at the side of the mouth or beak by the hinge of the jaw and gently introduce the liquid on the back of the tongue, a few drops at a time, allowing the patient to swallow without choking. Take great care with liquids: please read the section on 'Force-feeding' in Chapter 7 so that you are aware of the dangers and know what precautions need to be taken not to drown the animal. Chapter 7 also describes how to use a stomach tube, which might be necessary with some patients if all other methods fail.

Amphibians are much easier: they can absorb liquid doses through their skin if you add the medication to their vivarium water. Or give an oral dose by means of a syringe or stomach tube.

CHAPTER FOUR

SITUATIONS

ROAD TRAFFIC ACCIDENTS (RTAs)

Roads are battlefields for animals (as well as for some drivers) and RTAs probably account for more deaths and mutilations of animals like dogs, cats, foxes, badgers, deer, squirrels, rabbits and birds than almost any other single agent.

Slow-moving animals like hedgehogs and toads stand little chance against what is literally overhead traffic but it is surprising how often hedgehogs become walking wounded rather than flattened corpses, and it is usually worth making an effort to rescue them and restore them to health. Darting squirrels, never quite sure which way to jump, are more often killed outright. Nocturnal and crepuscular mammals like badgers, foxes and rabbits are common casualties, frequently hurt rather than killed, and will often drag themselves away from the road to lie up in a den, either to die slowly or to recover in due course. Cats, too, are common road casualties and also tend to crawl away into a ditch to die, the victims of hit-and-accelerate drivers who are more likely to stop and help an injured dog than a cat. Dogs allowed to roam by negligent owners are often either RTA victims themselves or are the cause of an accident, when drivers swerve to avoid them and, missing the dog (or not), collide with an oncoming car instead. Deer make their impact felt, but drivers either leave them where they lie injured or stop and do not know how to help.

Birds suffer considerable losses on the roads, especially in spring when the caterpillars from overhanging trees lie invitingly exposed on the tarmac or when unwary young birds have not yet learned how to judge the speed of the traffic.

If you come across (or are the cause of) an RTA victim, make sure you do not precipitate a worse accident by suddenly jamming on your brakes or swerving—which is the natural instinct. On no account stop on a motorway: the poor creature will quickly be put out of its misery under the wheels of the next few vehicles in moments. Act sensibly according to the business of the road and use your hazard warning lights when you do pull up. Then choose handling and first-aid techniques appropriate to the species, remembering always that the animal is likely to be frightened and therefore unnaturally aggressive, and will also need treatment for shock.

Park your vehicle between the animal and oncoming traffic if you can, and at night direct your headlights so that you can see and be seen. Never run to the animal's aid: for the sake of the victim and for the sake of bystanders, your whole attitude must be calm and reassuring throughout.

If the animal is still trapped under a vehicle or its wheels do *not* try and move the vehicle but jack it up carefully to release the animal, which might want to remain hiding underneath for security or from shock even if it is not badly injured.

Sometimes you will come across an animal at night which has simply been dazzled by headlights and only needs a chance to recover its night vision in darkness, which in the case of, say, an owl could take at least a quarter of an hour in a safe place. If you are driving at night, do watch out for badgers, deer and owls in particular, and if possible give them a chance to cross safely out of the way by stopping and turning off your lights.

When it is known that an animal has or might have been hit by a car but seems to have run off, do check nearby ditches, hedgerows and fields in case the creature is lying up with injuries and shock. Look out, too, for pets which escape from their owners' vehicles after an accident and run off in sheer panic and confusion. An animal might have to be tracked only a few yards or it might travel quite long distances, even if badly injured. In built-up areas, check under parked vehicles and sheds or in quiet, tucked-away corners, waste ground and derelict buildings; in the country follow natural highways like hedgerows—most animals, whether injured domestics or wild ones which are healthy or hurt, will avoid crossing open spaces and keep to the cover of the base of a wall or fence, or use the narrow tracks worn by generations of wild feet. Animals who know their area might well lie up near water, and sick ones will naturally choose somewhere dark and safe if they can reach it, though they might collapse in the open. Try and think yourself into the animal's mind; if your imagination needs help, read the tracking chapter in the NARA guide, *Animal First Aid,* or any good field guide for hunters and naturalists.

Remember that a person who has caused or witnessed an accident probably needs as much reassurance and consideration as the animal victim and might need treatment for shock themselves. If the owner of a domestic pet is present, do warn them that their pet could act with uncharacteristic violence even towards someone it knows, but it will make your job much easier if the owner is calm enough to help, and it makes the animal's chances of survival and recovery much higher if it is reassured by a familiar person when first approached. In general, a severely injured animal is easier to handle than one with minor injuries who is suffering more from fright than pain and will need restraint and reassurance.

As with all animal rescue situations, if you feel unable to deal with it yourself you should get hold of someone who can. For example, if a deer is injured in the road it usually needs more than one person to lift it carefully out of harm's way or into a vehicle, but it also needs handling by someone who understands deer. If, as so often happens, your car has hit a deer at night on a country road, get someone else to contact the police immediately while you stay with the animal. The police have plenty of experience of this situation and will be able to call up appropriate veterinary help or the RSPCA even if it is two in the morning, or can find a good shot with an appropriate weapon to put the deer out of its misery if that is the kindest course of action. If you feel justified in making a decision yourself about the advisability of ending the deer's life then and there, you could get in touch direct with a reliable local gamekeeper or perhaps a livestock farmer known to you. In some parts of the country there are "deer ambulance" services offered by wildlife rescue centres: the police will know of any local ones, or you can contact NARA, who have a 24-hour emergency service and have willing voluntary helpers on standby in several areas.

Drivers have a legal obligation to report to the police any accident involving dogs, cattle or horses but, even if there is no legal obligation, it is obviously considerate to make every effort to locate the owner of any domesticated animal and to leave final decisions on the animal's treatment to them once you have given all the help you can. It is the owner's right, for example, to choose which veterinary surgeon will treat the animal and sometimes a dog will wear an identification disc which gives a vet's name and telephone number as well as the owner's. Again, the police will help if ownership is not obvious; they are also likely to be better at breaking the bad news to a distressed owner and can probably arrange for the owner to be brought to the scene if transport is a problem. In addition they can handle traffic flow while the casualty is given first aid and of course deal with any damaged vehicle that has to be removed. The impact of a deer, for example, can result in a lot more than a dent to a car.

If a domesticated animal is already dead you should still do your best to inform its owner. There is nothing worse than worrying about the unknown fate of a missing pet.

In many cases a casualty is small enough for you to pick it up carefully and transport it for proper diagnosis and treatment, bearing in mind the relevant handling and first-aid techniques. As already described, such an animal can usually be wrapped in a jacket or sweater, both for warmth and restraint, and put on or under a car seat in darkness, but a cardboard box or a sack would give you more peace of mind if you are driving alone. Here are some of the items every car could carry, just in case:

> Cardboard box or sack (restraint, warmth, darkness)
> Old jacket, rug, sheet, groundsheet or towel (restraint, blanket stretcher, warmth)
> Improvised bandaging (clean handkerchieves, strips of clean sheet etc.)
> Rope
> Materials to improvise muzzles and other restraints (dog-lead, binder twine, neck tie)
> Gloves (strong enough to handle unwilling victims)
> Sharp knife (clean); wirecutters
> Torch
> Newspapers and plastic bags
> First-aid kit
> Bottle of water
> Road cones, hazard lights/signs, reflective waistcoat
> Crook, grasper, landing net, other nets
> Spade, crowbar

Another roadside hazard is strays, whether pets or livestock. If you find a lost-looking dog, for example, make sure that its owner is not in the immediate vicinity, perhaps taking it for a walk, before you bundle it into the car and take it to the address on the collar (where the owner will be out!) or to the local police or dog-rescue centre. It is worth asking about the animal's owner at, say, the local pub or garage or village shop before taking it out of the area.

Livestock should be shepherded off the road into the nearest field as a matter of urgency before there is an RTA. If the field contains a growing crop, the farmer will not be best pleased but that argument will be between the field owner and the livestock owner whose poor fencing allowed the animals to wander in the first place. Get plenty of help with the herding and make sure that all approaching vehicles have due warning of the hazard. Even narrow country lanes are regarded by some drivers as motorways and it is alarming how some of them resent slowing down at all even for a regular dairy herd which has used the road from field to milking-parlour for years.

A bolting horse can be very dangerous on the road, both to itself and to drivers. It will be in a state of panic. Make every effort to *stop* all traffic in both directions until the horse has either been caught or turned safely into a field or yard—and beware of the excited animal that leaps straight out of the field again over the fence. If the animal is wearing a saddle and/or bridle (the saddle might have come off in the meantime), there will be an injured or at least dazed or upset rider somewhere in the area and in need of help. Unless you have experience with horses, it is not sensible to stand in the path of an animal at full pelt.

TRAPPED

The pickles into which animals can get themselves are legion and in the great majority of cases it is the human hand that has put them there, directly or indirectly. The human race considers many species of living organisms to be its enemies and does its utmost to control or exterminate them, labelling as vermin, pests, weeds and so on, anything which competes with humans for living space and food.

But although we have filled the world with potential hazards, many of us care deeply about their consequences. If you are asked by other people to rescue any kind of living creature from any situation from which it cannot extricate itself, bear in mind the advice of the Guernsey SPCA to its wardens: "Any person telephoning us is asking for help, so please give it, however small the request. An injured sparrow is as important as an injured dog, cat or horse." In the context of birds stuck in chimneys, NARA puts it like this: "Elderly people care a great deal about small birds and if they believe that one has fallen down their chimney, they will turn off their heating which could, if not remedied quickly by the removal of the bird, lead in cold weather to the elderly person suffering from hypothermia."

Birds Indoors

If a bird enters a room, it tends to panic and fly against closed windows in its efforts to escape. Swallows in particular insist on remaining as close to the ceiling as possible, defying attempts to guide them to an open window only 6 inches below ceiling level. Draw all the curtains to darken the room and quieten the bird. Then either catch the bird, which is more easily done in darkness (drop a cloth over it if you wish) and release it outside, or draw back the curtain at an open window so that the bird is attracted to the escape route, provided that the whole light is open.

Bats found crawling vaguely in a room during the summer (or on a garden path) are likely to be lost babies. The indoor bat should be put in a ventilated box until near dusk, when it should be hung close to the roost entrance. The outdoor bat can be put back into the roost or nearby; put in an outbuilding until dusk or hung high on a tree trunk, wall or a similar position out of cat reach but accessible to the mother.

Chimneys

Birds in chimneys can be given the opportunity to escape into the room and then dealt with as above, but this is often impracticable. You might need to remove a false front from a blocked-off old fireplace, or to take out a heating installation. If it is a gas appliance, it is wiser to call the gas board to dismantle it safely than to do it yourself. If the chimney is sooty, the bird will need a gentle clean-up before it is released, especially around its eyes and beak. Make sure there are no injuries needing treatment and give the bird time to recover from shock in a warm, dark, quiet place.

Other creatures find themselves in chimneys, too—I know of at least one weasel which entered a room from the fireplace. A cat could, with skill, be rescued with the aid of a long pole (perhaps a set of drain rods) with a running noose at the end, but with cats and with larger birds like owls, which quite often find their way into chimneys, you will find that the fire brigade's animal rescue service is well equipped and helpful, though it should only be called upon when really necessary.

Holed Up

Sick or injured animals, wild or domesticated, often take refuge underground, whether in their own den or burrow, or under a shed or down a drainage pipe. Animals also put themselves into these situations by mistake: terriers get stuck down rabbit holes or (very dangerously for the dog) in a badger sett; pets fall down disused wells and shafts; hedgehogs tumble into uncovered stopcock pipes or down into the pits of cattlegrids or drained garden ponds; and ferrets are notorious for wilfully "lying up" in a warren.

An injured or sick animal which has gone to ground is more than likely to attack its rescuer if it cannot escape and you should approach and handle it with caution, as described in the various species-handling sections in Chapter 2. Wild mammals tend to squeeze themselves hard against the furthest end of their hiding hole, and sometimes wedge themselves more tightly by stretching their legs so that their backs are pressed against the top of the hole and it is very difficult to shift them. Try using a grasper to hold them around the neck while you use a crook to "walk" them towards you by drawing on their legs.

If a dog or ferret is down a burrow or den, it might be lost or involved rather than stuck. Try calling at the entrance hole or rattling a stick there to attract its attention and to guide a lost animal in the right direction. This might take quite a long time—hours, or even days—as some underground systems are large, rambling and confusing. Ferrets are usually good at finding their way out, in their own time: they might have killed a rabbit underground, gorged and gone to sleep after a good meal, and will come out in due course, probably several hours later when they are thirsty. Leave a familiar carrier by the entrance with a drink and some bedding, and no doubt the ferret will be curled up in it sound asleep when you come back the next morning.

If you do have to dig for an animal, take great care not to drive the spade straight into its skull or body! Dig carefully, by degrees. If the animal is wedged, it cannot evade your spade blade. However, to dig successfully you need to know a lot more about burrow systems and how to explore them, otherwise you will find yourself digging up half a field with no result. Use your *ears:* get down on your stomach, put your ear to the hole and listen, or use a "sounding stick"—a metal pole, with one end on the ground and the other against your ear—to check for vibrations underground. Be warned, however, that burrows ramble all over the place and the direction of a sound in such a system can become wildly distorted and deceptive.

A stuck animal, unless it is attacked by the local resident, can probably survive underground for quite a few days, during which time it will lose weight and thus might be able to free itself and escape of its own accord.

A hedgehog down a vertical standpipe can be difficult to get hold of: the pipe will be too long and narrow for your hands and the animal will be rolled up anyway, so that it soon becomes wedged. Use a pair of pliers: give the hedgehog some firm but kindly prods to encourage it to roll up even tighter, which makes it smaller, then carefully take hold of its back and quills with the pliers or grips and gently draw it free. However, you might have to dig out the whole pipe. In future, make sure the pipe is properly capped. Likewise, all pits like cattlegrids and empty ponds should be fitted with ramps to let hedgehogs escape, and if you find a hedgehog in a pit just put in a temporary ramp at as shallow an angle as possible and let it find its own way out.

Cats accidentally shut in buildings have been known to survive for up to six weeks without either food or water (they are a desert species and drink very little). If the cat is found unconscious, get veterinary assistance immediately because it will need intravenous drip-feeding. If it is conscious, introduce water and food *very* gradually: give it small amounts of water at a time, and do not give solids for the first three days but feed it on glucose or honey in water, milk (by itself or with a beaten egg yolk), Brands Essence, and Cimicat or a similar substance from the vet. After three days it can begin to eat small portions of poached white fish and gradually return to a normal diet.

Stranded

Animals, especially domestic pets, get themselves stranded up trees, on cliff-tops and ledges, and on roof-tops. Cats are said to climb anything when the wind (or a dog) is up their tails and often seem quite incapable of finding the way down again. Do not call the fire brigade for a high cat: the event is so frequent that the service is not allowed to respond unless the cat has been stranded for at least 72 hours, in which time it has often found its own way down anyway and is none the worse for the adventure.

Cat rescue from heights can be difficult and dangerous; it needs the right equipment and climbing skills as well as the knack of handling an irate cat. Talk to a friendly local tree surgeon, perhaps. Make sure that, once the cat is reached, it is caught with a landing-net and transferred securely into a sack to be lowered gently to the ground. Do not open the sack until it is in a confined space: a freed cat will quite probably shoot straight up the nearest tree again. Leave it alone in the confined space to recover its dignity and its nerves.

Cliff-tops and ledges are no places for inexperienced climbers either, however good they might be at animal rescue. Call in the trained rescue services. In extreme emergencies you could ask the coastguard or mountain rescue teams but remember that they are usually under pressure in saving human lives. Give the RSPCA, SSPCA or NARA a call to find your nearest animal rescue service or, if you happen to know them, try a mountaineering or pot-holing club, or voluntary groups that rescue climbers, cave explorers and fell walkers, or perhaps an off-duty post office or electricity board engineer used to climbing poles and well equipped with ladders, harnesses and ropes. Ask the local police for advice if necessary, or even the local paper if their contacts are good.

Wells and old shafts are also dangerous places for the amateur rescuer. You have only to think of some of the more infamous cases of well rescues to remember the frightening problems of collapsing sides and fatal falls. Do not risk the life of an inexperienced person as well as the animal victim, when an experienced, trained and properly equipped person could save themselves as well as the animal.

Ditches, Bogs and Slurry Pits

Livestock, especially cattle (who are wallowers by nature), can get themselves well and truly bogged down in an unprotected pitful of slurry, a cesspit or a marshy area. Cattle are quite capable of swimming but their own weight is their millstone in the quicksand-like suction of slurry and deep mud.

Farmers are often tempted to try and drag an animal out with the aid of a tractor hauling on a rope around the creature's neck but the animal is more likely to die as the result of such a "rescue" than it is to drown in the slurry in the first place. If at all possible, call the fire brigade and explain the situation: they are more than willing to help. Their animal rescue service will have proper equipment, techniques and experience for this quite common situation.

Two immediate problems are that the more the animal struggles, the deeper it is dragged down into the mire (slurry is often several feet deep), and the longer it is trapped the greater the restriction on the circulation of blood to its limbs. Each situation is unique but the fire brigade will probably use a combination of winches, tripods, body slings under chest and belly, and straw bales—the latter to give the animal something to scramble along in due course and in the meantime to help support its weight from underneath as the hoisting tackle does its work. It will be necessary to try and massage the animal's limbs to restore the circulation if they can be reached without the rescuer also becoming bogged down, and at the same time to try and remove the surrounding muck to free the limbs from the weight and give the animal a chance to use its own legs.

The whole operation needs to be given *plenty* of time and patience. At each stage the animal should be supported and allowed to rest, and kept warm with blankets. A crucial stage is when the animal first finds its feet on the straw-bale ramp (which needs to be as wide as possible). From this point, after due rest, it should be allowed to make its own way to firm ground, in its own time, with very gentle persuasion by means of a halter or by the pressure of a strap of webbing (or two people's linked arms) like a sling against its buttocks to heave it mildly forward.

Battling with a thick, viscous medium will exhaust the animal. Once it is safe, it will need to be rubbed down thoroughly to aid circulation as well as to clean off the very worst of the muck. Then it should be rugged for warmth and given a quiet, warm, private place to recover on good, fresh bedding, with access to ample drinking water and sweet hay. If you are sure it has not suffered any injury during its ordeal, a drink of strong tea might cheer it up, but not if it is going to need veterinary treatment. It would be wise to have a veterinary check anyway, just in case, especially with an in-calf cow.

Tangles

Sheep often get their fleeces tangled up in **brambles or fencing,** and in more remote areas they sometimes die slowly, caught in a thicket. Of course, the more they struggle the more entangled they become. They can also get themselves fouled up with fencing in their determined efforts to be on the greener side; in particular they will poke their heads through the large mesh of sheep-netting and then get a foot through another square, ending up in a tangle and a panic. The section on sheep handling in Chapter 2 gives advice for this sort of problem.

Tethered animals can get into very dangerous tangles if the basic rules for safe tethering are ignored. Goats in particular seem to be adept at hanging themselves from their own tethers and need urgent rescuing before they are throttled.

Railings of various kinds often trap animals, domesticated or wild, who, like children, get their heads wedged between two upright palings be they of sawn timber, split chestnut or iron. The occasional antlered deer who tries to get through too narrow a gap in this way can be in real trouble: its antlers prevent withdrawal, it panics, and the situation becomes terrifying. You need all your handling skills with this one, as well as tools capable of separating or cutting out the palings.

Barbed-wire—that barbaric stuff which the cattlemen of western America so deplored in frontier days and which is all too often the sign of a farmer whose hedges have been neglected—can cause horrifying injuries to animals in a panic.

Smaller animals, including cats and the smaller deer species, and numerous birds, especially kestrels and unsuspecting fledglings, become enmeshed in that fine green **nylon netting** which gardeners and fruit growers use to protect their plants and crops. Typically the victim dies a slow death, hopelessly trapped and unable to feed or drink, and also vulnerable to any passing predator, or it slowly strangles itself as the unforgiving filaments encircle its neck. At best, perhaps, the victim eventually struggles free, but it might have to rip off its foot to do so. Untangling the frightened victim takes considerable patience. In most cases it is best to cut out a whole segment of the mesh so that the animal is no longer part of the main netting, then work carefully with blunt-ended scissors to snip away the entanglement— every strand of it—paying special attention to the neck area to avoid asphyxiation. Because of the necessarily close contact with the frightened animal, you will have problems in restraining it while you work and you really do need another pair of hands to prevent the animal getting even more entangled in its efforts to escape from you. Remember that many creatures will be quieter if hooded or blindfolded.

Animals, and more specifically birds, get entangled in gardeners' seed-protecting **strands of cotton,** or in discarded **fishing lines,** and even in the trailing strings of a **kite.** A bird with a length of line snagged around its leg might fly off with the loose end trailing until the line catches like an anchor on a branch, a television aerial, a church spire or even a crane, and suddenly the bird is hanging upside-down in mid-air, well and truly trapped like a spring-caught hawk or snared mammal. Very often the situation needs a rescuer with climbing expertise to cut the line free from the gallows and bring the bird down to the ground so that it can be disentangled from its shackles. The bird needs to be checked for injuries: the line might have cut into the flesh, or damaged a wing so that its flying ability is impaired. If the line has become embedded, it will probably have interfered with the bloodflow to an extremity and there is the strong possibility of infection or even a need for amputation. Veterinary diagnosis and treatment are essential.

Fishing tackle can cause the most appalling suffering to waterfowl in particular, who not only get feet, bodies, wings, necks and beaks entangled in that fine, almost invisible, and defiantly non-biodegradable filament but also end up with fish hooks embedded in feet or bodies, or even halfway down the throat. For example, I have seen an innocent village-pond mallard gleefully taking a piece of bread off the water unaware that it was fishing bait, and swallowing the barbed hook along with the bread. In such a situation, or if you find a bird in obvious distress or looking underweight and poorly with a piece of fishing line hanging from its beak, do not cut off the loose end of the line because it might be a useful aid to the vet later, during the operation which might be needed to extract a hook from the throat or in the intestines. For advice on the removal of fish hooks see under 'Wounds' in the First Aid chapter.

Snares

Snares are deliberately set to kill. In theory they are set for specific species in controlled situations, are visited at least once every twenty-four hours (which is a long interval for an injured or dying victim) and are designed to kill instantly by strangulation. In practice, however, they are indiscriminate and very often catch quite a different species by the leg or body or muzzle so that it is trapped rather than killed outright. It might die a lingering death; it might struggle so frantically against the unrelenting wire that its flesh is severely injured; it might even in desperation chew off its own snared foot to escape. Snares catch rabbits and foxes by intent, and deer, badgers, cats, dogs and livestock by mistake, or mostly by mistake.

In theory, there are two types of snare: the free-running and the self-locking. With both types, the wire loop continues to tighten when an animal struggles to free itself, but a self-locking snare does not slacken off when the struggling is relaxed. It is now illegal under the Wildlife and Countryside Act 1981 to use a self-locking snare to take any wild animal but a free-running snare (see Fig. 9), which does slacken off, can legally be used to take any wild animal except those protected under the Act.

Many keepers still believe that self-locking snares are kinder if killing is deemed to be necessary, partly because it is easier to avoid catching the wrong species in a self-locking snare. The problem is that an unmodified free-running snare can easily become big enough to catch an animal around its body rather than its neck, and small enough to catch the leg of a deer unless the animal is deflected by a "deer leap"—a stout horizontal branch placed about 14 inches above ground level in front of the snare so that the deer is forced to leap over it safely.

If you do find a snared animal, act very fast before it can strangle itself. Take heed of the handling hints for the species and then get that snare off as quickly and efficiently as you can. Do not simply cut the wire between noose and peg, leaving the animal with the noose still around it, unless you have the animal so positively restrained that it cannot possibly escape until you have removed the noose. If the wire has cut into the flesh or constricted the blood supply, the animal will need veterinary attention. If the noose is around the animal's neck, *it is essential* to avoid inciting the animal to move suddenly or to try and pull away: it will be instantly throttled.

Traps

A spring trap has to be of an "approved" type under the WCA and the Act also lays down conditions governing where and when such traps can be used. In theory precautions must be taken to avoid catching birds, game or domestic animals. For example, it is not permissible to use an approved spring trap as a pole trap to catch a bird of prey landing on top of a post.

A properly sited and set spring trap should kill a specific pest instantly but many do not. Just like snares, they can catch an animal by its foot, causing excruciating pain and usually smashing the bones. Gin traps, which are spring traps with toothed jaws, have thankfully been banned for the last thirty years but an untoothed trap can be just as vicious. The other type of trap is the "live-catch", which might be anything from a cage with a trap door to a net. However, like snares, neither spring traps nor cage traps can be used to catch wildlife protected under Section 6 of the WCA.

Before releasing an animal caught by the leg in a spring trap, make quite sure you can restrain it so that its injuries and state of shock can be treated.

HUNTED

The main types of organised hunting in Britain are fox-hunting, cubbing, terrier work, beagling, harriers, hare-coursing, stag-hunting with hounds, deer-stalking, rifle shooting for larger game, shotgun shooting of game birds, wildfowling, rabbiting with the aid of dogs or ferrets and nets or lamps, rough shooting of either game or vermin (winged or otherwise), mink hunting (otter hunting is now illegal) and angling.

Then there are the illegal "sports" like badger-baiting, cock-fighting, dog-fighting and all sorts of poaching, the latter in our day being a high-tech business more likely to be for substantial profits than for the family pot. There are some good books covering the legal side of all these sports, legal and otherwise, listed in the Bibliography, and the League Against Cruel Sports (LACS) can give advice about taking legitimate action to deter hunts from entering prohibited land.

Whatever you think of the morality of various kinds of hunting, if it is legal you cannot legitimately interfere directly, but there are ways of making your point without breaking the law and, preferably, without incurring the hostility of those who do participate in the sport. Even with illegal sports, whatever your rights and moral obligations, you should be very wary of direct intervention. LACS advises that you should make no attempt to rescue a victim of badger-baiting or dog-fighting, however desperate its plight, but take a discreet note of vehicle numbers, make a rough description of the people and dogs involved, then get to the nearest telephone and dial 999 to report the matter to the police. The people involved in these sports are quite prepared to hand out more than verbal abuse to those they regard as their enemies.

Animal rescuers might be asked to deal with exhausted prey, savaged prey, injured prey like winged birds or animals which have been shot and abandoned but are not dead, and all sorts of victims of abuse like fighting dogs with their faces torn to ribbons, baited badgers with horrific injuries (read Chris Ferris's book *Out of the Darkness* if you can stomach it), severely lacerated fighting cockerels, and hounds electrocuted on railway lines or involved in RTAs—there is an endless list of the consequences of field sports. In the case of hounds, for those of you who might disagree with the hunters, do remember that their dogs are innocent and deserve the fullest sympathy and caring treatment of any animal rescuer.

If an exhausted hunted animal takes refuge in a house or vehicle in its desperation (and many chasing sports aim to exhaust their prey as much as outwit it), give it peace and security while it recovers; leave drinking water within its reach but do not try and approach or handle it, which would only cause more distress. However, if it has already been savaged it will obviously be in need of veterinary treatment. A hunted wild animal does not belong to the hunt, and if it is on your private property you have the right to protect it from further harrassment and fear.

ABUSED

This is a minefield. It is always advisable to get professional help if you come across what you think is a case of animal abuse. Those who actively abuse animals are equally capable of physically abusing you. There is also the problem of the law: for a start, do you have any right to take action yourself and, second, will your intervention in any case result in a prosecution?

If you do suspect active abuse contact the police, the RSPCA or an appropriate welfare or rescue group (see Chapter 11). There are special-interest groups for everything from hunt victims to battery hens and veal calves, and they have a lot more experience and influence than you do acting on your own.

There is also neglect of domesticated or confined animals—ill treatment by ignorance or carelessness rather than deliberate cruelty—and this, too, is best handled by the professionals, however heart-rending it might be to see a suffering animal.

If you find a stray animal, which might have been abandoned or might simply be lost, contact the police or take it to an appropriate rescue centre (dog home, cat home, donkey sanctuary etc.) but have the courtesy to telephone them in advance. If the animal does have a legal owner, you could unwittingly be guilty of theft if you keep the animal without making every effort to trace that owner. But you can make it clear that, should the real owner not be found or be unwilling to reclaim it, you would be glad to give it a home. However, the more responsible welfare groups need to satisfy themselves that the home you offer really is a good one and they will investigate your circumstances carefully. Do not be resentful or offended: they are acting in the animal's interest, which is more important than your own.

FIRE

Fire has always been a hazard for livestock and many are the tales of heroic people, and even heroic dogs, rescuing cattle, sheep, pigs and horses from burning farm buildings which, with plenty of hay and straw around the place, rapidly become death traps, killing by smoke inhalation as much as by burning. A poorly made haystack can combust spontaneously in certain conditions but most farm fires are probably caused by the careless disposal of cigarette ends, sparks from the workshop, children playing with matches among the straw bales or, sadly, by vandals and malicious arsonists.

Whenever you are faced with a fire in a building of any kind, whether agricultural or domestic, remember that smoke kills and that the admission of air dramatically accelerates the progress of a fire (for example, opening a door). Do not put your own life at risk, even for the sake of a distressed animal, because that will provoke a second person to risk their life to save yours. Let the experts handle it whenever possible.

However, in a desperate situation where pets or livestock are trapped, the golden rules are keep cool, keep your face covered, and keep as close to the floor as possible because smoke rises. Make sure that someone outside the building knows you are in there so that you can be rescued yourself if overcome by fumes (it helps if you are linked by a rope so you can be pulled out). Naturally the owner of the farm building should be alerted and the emergency services contacted. If time permits, ask how many animals are housed, and where within the building if its layout is not obvious.

Any animal in a burning building will be terrified and could be difficult to handle. If there are only one or two animals, use blindfolds to calm them as you lead or carry them to safety, and if you are removing a small animal through a broken window do cushion the jagged lower edges with a jacket so that the animal is not accidentally lacerated. With livestock it is preferable to release them methodically from their stalls and let them find their own way out. Keep well clear of the escape door or the stampede could flatten you.

Horses are generally more highly strung than other livestock and have been known to rush back into a blazing building simply because it is a place they know and within which they feel safe.

Any animal which has been trapped is likely to be in a severe state of shock even if it has escaped being burned. First aid should therefore concentrate on keeping the animal reassured, quiet and warm, unless there are burns which you feel competent to treat until the vet arrives. Remember that the immediate need is to reduce the heat of the seared flesh.

Forest and heath fires are rarely so sudden and rapid that wildlife cannot escape but slow-moving animals such as toads could be in bad trouble. If you see any that are literally in the line of the fire, grab them and run to a place of safety. Quite often, however, and surprisingly, these fires are superficial in that they remove vegetation but scarcely touch the ground itself, so that burrowing animals might be perfectly safe. At the first sign of a fire in such open spaces, alert the emergency services even before you start taking action yourself: the sooner they can arrive, the greater their chance of controlling the spread of the fire. Then alert any livestock owners in the area so that they can move their animals to safety if necessary, and keep a sharp eye out for very young animals like calves and fawns which might be lying up and will automatically stay just where they are rather than make a run for it.

DROWNING

Just about any animal can swim, instinctively, even if it is very young, and many are quite strong swimmers. Even a cat can swim if it must, and likewise a ferret which would not voluntarily take a dip for pleasure. Problems arise if the water is very cold, if the animal has to struggle in strength-draining mud or becomes entangled in its own halter or lead or in submerged vegetation, if the sides of the watercourse impede exit or the animal panics and swims away from the shore, or if the weight of wet fleece or fur causes exhaustion. Sheep seem to be particularly susceptible to drowning: most of them hate swimming anyway, and a wet fleece can double their weight in no time. Cattle, on the other hand, have been known to swim considerable distances (even miles) and their short coats do not hinder their efforts, though neither do they give good insulation. Pigs swim too, despite the old wives' tale about them cutting their own throats with their trotters when they paddle. Horses sometimes swim for pleasure (there was a famous one in the nineteenth century which would leave its stable of its own accord on many a morning to wander down to the beach for a dip).

There are many stories of heroic rescuers saving drowning animals (and equally of heroic animals saving drowning people). If you do decide to swim to the rescue, try and find a rope so that you have a lifeline to the bank and can haul yourself back to safety. Of course, if there is a boat to hand, use it, preferably with two people, and beware of overturning the vessel as you lean over the side to pick up a thrashing animal. Or get some kind of improvised raft under the animal to help it float—perhaps a plank or a lifebuoy.

If the water is very cold, an immersed rescuer will only remain of practical use to the animal for perhaps two minutes, and will be unconscious after four, but in summer a strong swimmer could remain active for perhaps twenty or thirty minutes. Take off boots, shoes and heavy jackets, but keep on other clothing, including socks, for insulation.

A submersed animal will be asphyxiated after about four minutes and will die, but over a shorter period do not be deceived into assuming it is dead:

it might only collapse and appear dead but can be resuscitated. If an animal was already badly injured when it entered the water and was thus unable to swim, it needs very urgent rescuing indeed: its specific gravity will be slightly greater than that of water, so that it will immediately submerge.

If the banks are steep, it will need at least two people to lift an animal from the water—one in the water with the animal to take its weight from below and the other on the shore. Watch out for crumbling banks, especially the deceptive kinds where the water or burrowing animals have eroded them out of sight below the waterline.

In the case of, say, a horse or large dog which has fallen into a swimming pool (probably one covered by a tarpaulin) and cannot scramble out because of the pool's vertical sides, provide the animal with an escape ramp with the gentlest possible slope or throw in some weighted straw bales as stepping stones, before the endless swimming completely exhausts the animal.

A rescued animal might appear unconscious or even dead, but do not give up hope of saving its life. As described in the First Aid section, the first and most urgent task is to get the water out of its lungs. Act fast, especially if the animal has been in the water for a while. The next step is to keep the animal's mouth open and give artificial respiration, and cardiac massage if necessary. As soon as possible' thereafter, get the animal dry by rubbing with a rough towel (which will also encourage blood circulation) and keep it in a warm place as you would any shocked patient. Give a large animal adequate rugging, and a smaller one would also benefit from hot-water bottles. Hypothermia and pneumonia are two strong possibilities after such an incident unless you take every step to keep the animal warm, quiet and reassured. Some animals, especially dogs and pigs, might also suffer from salt poisoning if they have swallowed sea-water.

ICE

The rescue of a drowning animal is greatly complicated if the water has iced over. You have very little time indeed to save the animal, not so much from drowning, perhaps, as from hypothermia. Very cold water kills. However, stop and think before you act.

The most likely victims of falling through ice on a pond are dogs, and their problem is that they cannot get a grip on the ice to lever themselves out of the hole. You have two main choices: go out to the animal over the ice, or go out through it. The former is preferable unless there is a boat or raft: do not put your own life at risk by wading through icy water unless you really have no option.

Tie a rope under your arms and either tie the other end to a tree or give it to someone on the shore (or on skates, if they lie on their stomachs and grip the surface of the ice with skate-tips) so that you can be hauled back to safety if the ice cracks under your weight. The art with ice is to spread your weight over the widest possible area rather than concentrating it all in your feet. Lay a plank or ladder or pole across the ice and use it as a bridge. Cautiously edge your way towards the animal and, as you near the hole, lie flat on your stomach to spread your weight as you actually effect the rescue.

A small dog will be relatively easy to pull out and carry back to the shore (again, go cautiously to avoid cracking the ice) but something the size of a labrador will be heavy and awkward. Each situation will be different and you will need to use your commonsense and ingenuity.

If there is a boat nearby, use it, or improvise a wooden sledge or stretcher of some kind which can be slid out over the ice and can still keep you out of the water if the ice should crack. In either case try and have a rope as a lifeline back to the shore.

If there is no equipment at all, you will have to smash your way through the ice but that is very much a last resort. Remember that a fit person will only remain effective in chilly water for about two minutes.

Waterfowl are less likely to trap themselves in ice, though people are often fooled by birds which are in fact merely resting on top of it. NARA's method of checking on the numerous reports of trapped winter birds (and 95 per cent prove to be false alarms) is for two people to walk on opposite banks dragging a long rope between them over the ice until, very gently, the rope nudges the suspect bird. If it is not trapped, it will stand up or be slid gently along the surface, but if it does not move, it cannot, and it needs to be rescued. The rope can also be used to rescue a swan which has landed so heavily on ice that it has sprained a leg: gently and carefully slide the big bird towards the shore by using the rope as a sweeper.

An animal rescued from an ice-hole will need immediate treatment to guard against hypothermia and shock. A bird will need to remain in a warm place for at least twelve hours before it is released again.

HIBERNATION

Most of our native amphibians and reptiles and a few mammals hide up somewhere safe in the winter and conserve their energy at a time when food is in short supply. Some of these are true hibernators: their bodies undergo quite drastic physiological changes with a warm-blooded animal becoming cold-blooded—literally—and they are easily mistaken for dead because their bodies feel so cold; in addition their heart beats and breathing are barely detectable and very, very slow.

Bats become periodically torpid from perhaps October to April. Before the cold weather comes, many increase their bodyweight by up to 35 per cent to see them through the months when their insect diet is likely to be lean. While hibernating they react to changes of temperature in their environment and can, slowly, awaken enough to change their quarters if necessary. They prefer humid conditions in their hibernacula, and if they do need to move they also need to have a drink.

Hedgehogs find themselves a dry nest, perhaps under tree roots or compost heaps and sheds, or down a rabbit hole or in a bramble patch. They are not true hibernators: they wake up quite often, even if they do not bother to come out of their nest. Hedgehogs, like bats, are insectivores and their food is in short supply in winter, but they have more catholic tastes than do bats.

The only native rodent in Britain which is a true hibernator is the dormouse, and it will be completely inactive for most of the winter, only beginning to stir in the latter part of its hibernation. Squirrels, contrary to popular lore, do *not* hibernate: they are usually active and out and about for a while on almost everyday of the year.

SNOW

Every year, drifting snow buries sheep which have perhaps taken shelter in the lee of a wall or hedge. Under its blanket the animal will be warm and snug, and as long as it has a breathing space it will not come to much harm, usually emerging much more fit than its rescuers expected even after several days under the snow. Do dig very cautiously: the sheep will not be able to move when you drive the spade blade down into the snow. A handling crook and a dog with a good nose could be useful.

ON THE FARM

No farmer can be with the livestock twenty-four hours a day and accidents do happen on even the best managed farms, especially where grazing is a long way from the farmstead. Sometimes a farmer will resent interference but more often there will be gratitude for an extra pair of eyes and hands to spot and help an animal in distress. Typical emergency situations, apart from entanglements and boggings, are a sheep on its back (see Chapter 2:

'Sheep'), difficult births (see 'Parturition', below), and bloat.

Bloat is a condition in which a ruminant animal's rumen (one of its stomachs) blows up with gas like a balloon when for some reason the animal has not been able to release normal rumen gases by means of belching and so on. Bloat can kill. If you see a ruminant (cattle, sheep, goats) with only its left-hand side blown up big and tight, send for the farmer and in the meantime keep the animal moving about if it is still on its feet, but do not cause it undue stress.

Emergency remedies for bloat include peanut oil (a pint in warm water for cattle), liquid paraffin (50 ml for a goat), washing soda crystals (for cattle, ¼ lb dissolved in hot water then diluted to about a pint with cold) and numerous country recipes known only to those who use them. These remedies are given as a drench, but only if you know how. Whatever the term implies, a drench is not a dowsing but is a method of getting liquids into the stomach quickly by pouring them gently down the animal's throat. There is a risk of drowning the animal by pouring liquid into its lungs by mistake.

Another possible emergency at pasture is the sight of sheep or cattle staggering about the field in spring and then collapsing. Very urgent help is needed for a condition known colloquially as **staggers** or more technically as hypomagnesaemia (magnesium deficiency) but there is nothing you can do yourself except alert the farmer or a vet, who will give the animal an immediate intravenous injection of magnesium salts. The animal is likely to be highly excitable and nervous, and needs very careful handling indeed.

PARTURITION

Very occasionally you might come across a farm animal in labour and in distress. Obviously you should alert the farmer immediately but there might be times when you need to give help on the spot. However, do not try and help with a birth unless you know what you are doing, and even then do not be too eager to interfere with the birth unless it is essential to do so.

There are perhaps two main problems you might encounter in the field: the foetus is wrongly presented in the womb so that it finds difficulty in leaving the mother's body, or the mother might be wandering around several days later with the afterbirth hanging out or, more rarely, with a prolapsed uterus which, to the layman, might look similar.

Be prepared to lend a hand under the farmer's guidance if you have given warning of a difficult birth. You will probably be asked to pull carefully on a rope tied to a stuck calf's fetlocks, making sure you do so in time with the cow's own contractions. Sheep seem to be more likely than cows to have problems with birth and many lambs seem to be determined to die whereas calves are determined to live. If you come across a newly-born animal whose mother is ignoring it or is incapable of attending to it, make sure it can breathe: wipe the birth fluids from its nostrils and mouth, and precipitate its first breath if necessary by tickling the inside of its nostrils with a straw. An abandoned or orphaned new-born needs special attention, and quickly, with top priority being given to warmth and massage.

It is quite normal for a herbivore mother to eat her own **afterbirth,** both to reabsorb useful nutrients and to clear away evidence of the birth so that predators are not alerted. However, the mother sometimes fails to eject the afterbirth completely within a normal period of, say, three or four days, and she wanders around with it trailing behind her. Do *not* try and yank it free yourself; this could do irreparable internal damage to the animal and render her incapable of reproduction.

The afterbirth is thin and stringy, but if what is hanging out of the animal is heavy, bulky and red, then she is suffering from a **uterine prolapse** and quick action is needed. It is an emergency and the vet should be summoned; in the meantime the animal needs to be restrained and confined, and you must try and keep the everted uterus clean and undamaged until the vet can push it back into its proper place.

BEACHED

Expert help is essential in dealing with beached cetaceans (whales, dolphins and porpoises). Someone should immediately be sent to contact the local RSPCA/SSPCA and a good vet, the coastguard and the police, and possibly the fire brigade. In the meantime, keep dogs and people well out of the way: be quite firm about this, for the sake of the onlookers, as there is some risk of physical danger and perhaps disease, and also for the animal itself. Beached animals are already under stress and too often die for that reason: they are wild animals in a totally alien environment, and they need peace and quiet, with no alarming noises or sudden movements. They also need reassurance and it can help if you talk gently and caress the animal. Do take care, however: a dying cetacean is likely to be thrashing about helplessly and by virtue of its size it could knock you flying with its tail.

Do not panic while you wait. Cetaceans are not fish: they can survive out of water for some time if you take certain precautions. They can breathe on dry land, albeit uncomfortably. However, their breaths are always well spaced out: dolphins and porpoises take a breath perhaps once every thirty to sixty seconds, and some of the whales might only take one breath in twenty minutes. The out-breath is explosive (hence the blow-hole jet when the animal has been underwater) and is followed very quickly by the intake, after which the blow-hole is covered by its flap until the next breath. But an unconscious animal stops breathing, because the act of breathing for these marine creatures is a conscious rather than reflex action.

It is vital to keep the beached animal's blow-hole clear so that it *can* breathe, and if possible it should be kept on its belly for that reason. However, it will probably be lying on its side when it is found, and needs to be carefully rolled over without damaging the flippers. Do not drag it by the tail while trying to get it upright as that will damage its spine. It would be best to wait for professional help, but if you can prop the animal up in the meantime, do so. A big animal will need the assistance of the fire brigade's jacking equipment, and it might be necessary to dig a pit to retain the animal's upright position in due course.

It is also important to keep the animal's skin cool and wet, without getting any water into the blow-hole (which would choke and drown it). Dowse it with cold sea-water until the firemen arrive; also use wet cloths and seaweed to cover it, and keep its eyes bathed if possible.

It is absolutely essential to keep the animal cool. If the sun is hot, shade must be provided to protect the skin from drying and blistering. The skin is so delicate that even a finger-nail can scratch it, yet these animals often recover from quite severe flesh wounds.

If the experts, when they arrive, consider that refloating should be attempted, it is sensible to wait for the tide to come up to the animal, though a small one can be carried by one or two people down to the water. A larger animal would need to be carried in a blanket stretcher (never drag any animal to the sea) and this will be necessary if conditions are such that you cannot wait for the tide—for example, it is very hot or the weather is bad. You should not, of course, take these decisions yourself unless you have plenty of experience, nor should a beached cetacean be moved until it has been examined by an expert.

Your work is by no means over when the animal is in the water. It needs to be held so that it can reorientate itself, and it should also be rocked from side to side to massage its stiff muscles and restore the circulation. You might need to remain with the animal for several hours in the water until it is fully recovered and ready to leave. A small animal can be kept in the shallows for this rehabilitation, just touching the ground but with most of its weight supported by the water; take it into deeper water now and then to see if it will swim off, otherwise bring it back to the shallows for more rocking. Once an animal is capable of floating and is willing to swim, escort it seawards with divers and small boats. But before then, take the opportunity of the long hours of closeness to take note of any distinguishing features on the animal so that it can be recognised later. If it persistently strands itself something is very wrong.

Cetaceans need sea-water but they can just about survive in **fresh water** for up to about two weeks, by which time irregular pale patches appear on their bodies as the upper layers of skin are lost. If an animal has lost its way up a river or canal, it needs to be carefully and gently guided back to the sea by boats. It is very likely to panic if put under stress, so that the whole manoeuvre must be well planned and carried out without haste or sudden activity. A panicky animal is likely to dive under the shepherding boats and head further upstream.

OIL AND POLLUTION

The increasingly prevalent problems of pollutants, many of which are insidious in their effects, cause widespread distress to wildlife. In the context of this book animal rescuers will be concerned with obvious and immediate emergencies involving fossil-fuel products like oil and tar.

The initial handling and first-aid treatment of a victim of pollution can be crucial to the success of subsequent treatment and its long-term well-being, so, in addition to the information given below, please bear in mind all the relevant principles outlined in earlier sections. In the case of oiled birds, the second stage—that is, cleaning, nursing and subsequent rehabilitation—is best carried out by those with considerable technical experience. Nevertheless some detailed information on dealing with oiled birds is given in Appendix 1, partly to deter amateurs from making a mess of it all and partly to encourage as many people as possible to become more professional so that they really can help rather than hinder in major rescue operations. No techniques can be described as absolutely correct or flawless and any method will have its critics, but it is hoped that the notes in Appendix 1, which rely on the considerable experience of the RSPCA, will be accepted as more sensible and practical than some.

Water-soluble Contaminants

Remove as much as you can with tissues then wash with plain water. Do not add detergents: they increase the wetting power of water and thus increase the skin's ability to absorb the contaminant.

Tar

Tar is often found on beaches where people, dogs and other unwary creatures get it on their feet or other parts of the body. To remove manageable amounts of tar from, say, a dog's paws or a cat's fur, use household margarine, melted butter, eucalyptus oil or Swarfega.

Creosote

Wash off creosote as soon as possible, using plenty of warm, soapy water or try warm castor oil. Clip off some of the hair if necessary so that you can clean the skin thoroughly.

Anti-perching Jelly

Try using biodegradable marine detergent to remove anti-perching jelly (used to deter pigeons from making a mess of public buildings). It is non-toxic and can also be used to remove oil from skin or plumage, but it is expensive and it is quite difficult to remove the residues of the cleaner, so that it is not advisable to use it on the plumage of any waterfowl or seabirds.

Oiled Birds

There are two major direct effects of oil pollution on birds. Externally, feathers clogged with oil are no longer effective in their vital functions of insulation and waterproofing: the bird loses body heat and buoyancy, and either loss can be fatal. A seabird depends on being able to rest on the sea and to dive for food, and lack of buoyancy inhibits both these essential abilities.

Then there is the very dangerous and likely possibility that the bird will ingest some of the oil in its attempts to preen it off its plumage. It might also ingest the emulsifying agents which are often spread to disperse oil slicks. If oil has been ingested, the bird's droppings will be yellow and it needs a good dose of liquid paraffin to help absorb some of the oil from the gut walls and get it out of the bird's system a little more quickly. However, there is a danger that fat-soluble vitamins (especially Vitamin A) will also be absorbed and lost, therefore the bird's diet will very probably need vitamin supplements.

Any treatment of an oiled bird must therefore deal with both external and internal pollution; but the bird must first be caught and it is likely that it will already be weak from its inability to feed and rest and perhaps from frantic preening efforts. The stress of capture is likely to be so considerable that on no account should the additional stress of the washing process follow immediately after capture. The bird must be given a chance to rest in warmth and peace; shock is a more immediate problem than oil. Let us therefore start at the beginning.

Capture   This is covered in the section on bird handling in Chapter 2. If possible—and without doubt if a lot of birds are in trouble—contact the experts to deal with the situation. Both the RSPCA and SSPCA have specialist oiled-bird units and can be contacted through your local society.

Immediate care   Put the rescued bird in a warm, dark container: a large, clean cardboard box with adequate ventilation holes is ideal. Do not use any straw, hay or other dry, dusty materials for bedding as they often contain fungi which can cause aspergillosis, a respiratory infection to which seabirds are especially vulnerable.

Try and leave the bird in absolute peace for a while to recover from the stress of capture and keep warm. Do not make any attempt at all to clean it at this stage: you must avoid additional stress until the bird is stronger. Certainly do not try dusting it with talcum powder, which will make it much more difficult to remove the oil later.

In the meantime, contact the nearest specialist oiled-bird cleaning and rehabilitation centre, who will give advice on preparing the bird for transportation. Resist the temptation to keep checking on the bird unless you can do so without it being aware of you: the less human contact it has, the better its future chances.

Transport   Birds can be safely transported in their cardboard boxes or in the type of pet boxes supplied by veterinary surgeons. Two or three birds of the same species can be put into the same box if it is big enough, and any flock bird would probably appreciate the company of its own kind, but do not mix the species and try to avoid mixing different sizes together. Keep the birds in darkness to keep them calm on the journey. Do not put them in plastic or polythene sacks, and do make sure that they can become neither chilled nor overheated: they should not be too crowded.

Larger birds such as swans and geese can travel loose in a van as long as their wings are strapped down in some way to prevent them flapping about and damaging either themselves or someone else.

Feeding   Food is a secondary consideration, though the birds will need feeding if there will be a delay of more than a couple of hours or so before the birds are able to reach a proper cleaning station. It is important to offer food appropriate to the species, and the food must be very, very fresh or, if frozen, it should be recently thawed. Your first problem, therefore, is to identify the species of bird accurately, which can be difficult with the younger ones, and then to find out as much as possible about its normal requirements and behaviour patterns.

Cleaning   An oiled bird stands a far greater chance of a successful return to its natural habitat if it is cleaned by those with considerable experience, who will not only clean the bird but will also ensure that its plumage is restored to perfect condition before it is eventually released in the right environment for its needs, at the right time. There is very little point in subjecting a wild bird to all the traumas of close handling that are unavoidable during a thorough cleaning operation, only to release it in the wild quite unfit to survive. Too many birds are released with the balance of natural plumage oils and feather structure so inadequate that they very quickly drown, or suffer from lack of insulation, or become incapable of feeding and die slowly. It is better to transport a bird for quite long distances for appropriate care than to make a mess of its life yourself.

If you happen to live on an island and have no means of transporting an oiled bird to the mainland for expert cleaning, or you are interested in learning the procedure, the basic essentials are given in Appendix 1.

DISEASES

It is comparatively rare to come across diseased wild creatures: they tend to show few symptoms until it is too late to help, and they hide themselves away. How often have you found the body of a wild animal which has died of natural causes, if ever? Symptoms are usually no more than a general disinterest and loss of condition which, unless you know the individual already, you are unlikely to notice.

Any wild creature which is obviously sick is probably very ill indeed and possibly close to death, especially if you are able to catch it. If you suspect disease of any kind, take sensible precautions to protect yourself and to avoid spreading the disease to healthy animals. Isolate the animal until you know what is wrong with it; wear gloves to handle it, wash your hands thoroughly anyway; scrub all utensils and tools and sterilise them before they are used for any other animal, and be aware that you could transmit an infection from one animal to another by means of your clothes and footwear as well.

Above all, consult a vet for professional diagnosis and advice on treatment and accommodation. However clever you are at nursing animals, you do need to know exactly what the problem is before you can deal with it successfully.

CHAPTER FIVE

KIND KILLING

There will be cases when a decision has to be taken to end a suffering animal's life. For many people, that decision poses considerable moral and practical dilemmas, and if possible it should be taken in consultation with a veterinary surgeon, who can then quickly and humanely put the animal to sleep so that its suffering is over. However, some vets are still tempted to advise euthanasia rather than struggle to keep an animal alive and help it to recover.

The Universities Federation for Animal Welfare (UFAW), in *Humane Killing of Animals* (which should be on every wildlife rescuer's bookshelf), suggests that typical situations in which kind killing might be necessary include animals suffering severe and unrelievable pain (for example, the effects of deadly poisons) or severe injury with no hope of recovery, or a case in which an animal is so vicious that it represents a danger to others. You also need to be aware of the laws which protect certain wild species from being killed except by licence (see Chapter 10).

If you are dealing with a domesticated animal, the decision must be the owner's, preferably in consultation with a vet, and the animal will in most cases be reassured by the owner's presence as long as that person is able to remain calm and comforting. Always get a qualified person to end the life of a domestic pet, however dramatic the situation might be, and always do exactly what the expert tells you to do, or you are no help at all.

It can be difficult to judge whether an animal *is* in severe pain. Some people claim that the "lower order" animals have little or no experience of pain or fear, but how do they know? It can be even more difficult to assess whether or not an animal's injuries are so severe that it will never recover, or whether it has suffered some permanent disability that will make it dependent on humans for the rest of its life. For example, birds of prey rely on their eyesight when hunting. A blind hawk clearly cannot survive except in captivity but a one-eyed bird, which you might think would be unable to judge its target with enough accuracy to catch a meal, can eventually adapt to its disability just as a person learns to adapt. The bird's problem is getting enough nourishment to keep it alive and fit while it is adjusting its skills.

The methods of compassionate killing outlined below are the quickest and most humane, as recommended by UFAW, and Appendix 2 suggests, in order of preference, the methods most suitable for each species. Once the decision has been taken, the act must be carried out with the least possible fear and suffering for the animal, and that means either instant death before it is aware of any threat, or instant unconsciousness so that it is unaware of the killing. An animal is not truly dead while its heart is still beating or its brain still functioning, even if it is not breathing, and it is essential to make quite certain that it *is* in fact dead. After death, the muscles at first relax completely; they gradually stiffen as rigor mortis sets in and then relax again after anything up to 48 hours.

The most aesthetic method of killing is very often *not* the most humane and if you have any qualms at all about either making the decision or carrying out the deed, do not do it. You will only make a mess of the whole business and could cause great distress to the animal. If the situation is not appropriate for a vet, find someone else with experience of humane killing—a gamekeeper, a police officer, a poultry farmer, an RSPCA inspector, a licensed slaughterer, a pest control officer or a wildlife hospital. Remember at all times to do what is best for the *animal*.

In the case of RTAs involving birds or small mammals immobilised and crushed beyond repair, the quickest solution is to drive your vehicle so that the wheels deliberately and accurately run over the victim's head and chest, killing the poor creature instantly. This method gets over the problem of direct contact with the animal which many people prefer to avoid.

In theory there is always a choice of physical methods, usually rather less crude than squashing an animal under your tyres, or chemical methods such as gas inhalation or an overdose of anaesthetics, but in practice the latter are under veterinary control. If you have to deal with a situation yourself, you are more likely to use physical methods of killing, especially in the case of, say, an RTA in the middle of nowhere in the middle of the night. Here you will probably have to resort to using your own hands to break an animal's neck, or use the nearest heavy object to stun and kill it, if mercy killing is necessary.

Shooting

The use of firearms is for those with licences and expertise only. These weapons are used to kill instantly with the first shot, which means that the aim must be accurate and correct (see Figs. 25–32 for the point of aim for various species). Use soft-nosed or hollow-nosed rifle bullets for preference. If in doubt about the result of the shot, shoot again or bleed the animal (see 'Exsanguination' below). In urban areas you should seek police permission before shooting.

POINTS OF AIM FOR CAPTIVE BOLTS AND FREE-BULLET PISTOLS

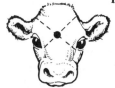

FIG. 25   CALF

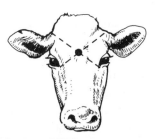

FIG. 26   COW
For bulls and heavy-boned animals, aim half an inch to side of thick bony mid-line.

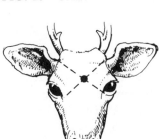

FIG. 27   DEER

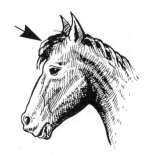

FIG. 28   HORSE
Aim high on forehead just *above* point where imaginary lines cross between opposite eyes/ears.

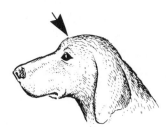

FIG. 29 DOG
Aim slightly to one side of mid-line to avoid bony plate.

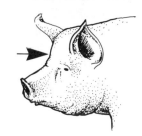

FIG. 30   PIG
Aim at point on mid-line 1 inch above eye level.

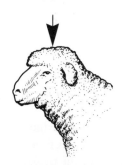

FIG. 31   SHEEP

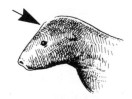

FIG. 32   SEAL

Stun Weapons

An alternative to shooting is the use of either a humane slaughtering free-bullet pistol typically used by vets and licensed horse slaughterers, or a captive-bolt pistol, another type of humane killer which fires an automatically recoiling bolt into the brain. Using the right bolt and technique, some animals can be killed outright by this weapon if the bolt penetrates deep into the brain, but others will only be stunned and should collapse instantly, with some involuntary thrashing of the limbs. To ensure death, slit the unconscious animal's throat to sever the main blood vessels.

Stun/Kill

This method is only for the self-assured and resolute: to be humane it must be done with determination, strength and speed. The aim is to stun the animal with a sharp, heavy blow to the back of the head so that it is knocked unconscious by the first impact, then to immediately make quite sure of its death while it remains unconscious, by repeating the blows as necessary or by neck-breaking, decapitation or asphyxia. A sufficiently damaging and accurate first blow can kill instantly by destroying the brain or severing the spinal cord. The stun/kill method can be used on a wide variety of animals, ranging in size from a small calf or an RTA dog to a small bird, rodent, amphibian or reptile. The techniques are as follows:

(1) Take a heavy, blunt instrument of a suitable size for the animal—whatever is to hand. For example: spanner, brick, spade, heavy stick, angler's "priest", baseball bat, poultry stunner. Bring it down sharply and hard at the back of the animal's head. With a hedgehog, however, aim for the top or front of the head instead.

(2) Alternatively, hold the animal by its back legs and swing it very hard so that the back of its head strikes something solid and hard-edged like a table, rock, gatepost, tree, sink or wall.

Neck-breaking (Cervical Dislocation)

This is probably the quickest and thus kindest mercy-killing method for **smaller animals** which can be easily handled, but you *must* have ample practice on dead animals first. The aim is to destroy the brain by severing the spinal cord.

(1) Hold the animal head down by its hind legs. Use the bony edge of your hand, or a blunt instrument, to deliver a sharp karate chop accurately on the vulnerable spot at the joint between the back of the neck and the cranium. This should only be done by those with experience, for

example, ferreters and gamekeepers. If you are dealing with a tough-necked old hare, the blow will hurt your hand and probably fail to kill the animal: use a blunt instrument.

(2) Hold the animal head down by its hind legs. With the other hand take the top of its neck between the vice of two fingers, or thumb and finger, palm outwards. Push that hand down while pulling up on the legs with the other, to stretch the animal's neck, and at the same time turn its head backwards at a right angle and jerk sharply downwards so that you feel (or hear) the dislocation (see Fig. 33). There will be instant loss of consciousness and rapid death, though the animal might flutter and jerk involuntarily for a few minutes. You need long arms and strength for this technique, particularly with a long-necked duck or a big hare.

(3) Put a **small rodent** or shrew on a flat surface (table top) and hold it by the tail. It will automatically try and pull away from you. Press a pencil or stick over its neck close to the head and then pull firmly until you feel the neck break (see Fig. 34).

NECK DISLOCATION

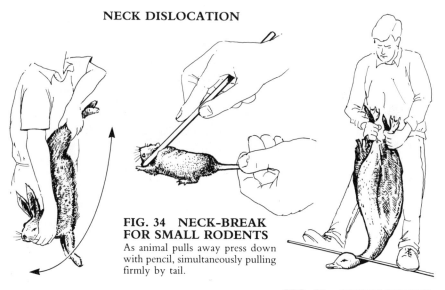

FIG. 34 NECK-BREAK FOR SMALL RODENTS
As animal pulls away press down with pencil, simultaneously pulling firmly by tail.

FIG. 33   POULTRY AND RABBITS
Pull hands apart to stretch neck while pushing chin up and back to dislocate.

FIG. 35   BROOMSTICK METHOD FOR LARGER FOWL
Brace your weight on broomstick while pulling bird's legs upwards to dislocate neck.

(4) A similar method can be used for a **heavy bird** like a goose. Hold the bird by its legs and wings in both hands and let its head and neck rest on the ground. Get an assistant to put a stout broomstick across the neck

near the back of the head, then put your feet on either end of the stick and use your whole weight to anchor the bird while you pull its body sharply upwards to dislocate the neck (see Fig. 35).

(5) With a small, fragile animal like a **bat,** rest it on a hard flat surface, put a pencil or stick across the back of its neck and press firmly to crush the vertebrae and break its neck.

(6) For **poultry, game and other large birds,** use either a bloodless castrator or a Semark game dispatcher, which crushes the spinal cord and blood vessels without breaking the skin or decapitating the bird. In the field, many game shooters despatch a wounded heavy bird by grasping its head and then swinging it around vigorously a couple of times with a quick jerk upwards or sideways in mid-swing to dislocate the neck.

(7) **Chicks** and **small birds** can be held by the body in one hand and by the head in the other; twist to break the neck.

(8) With unconscious **fish,** put your finger or a pencil in its mouth and then pull the head back sharply and decisively until the spine breaks.

Decapitation

This might seem to be the kindest cut of all but unfortunately it is not. (It can also be extremely messy: blood spurts out strongly.) A conscious animal is thought to remain conscious after decapitation for perhaps half a minute in the case of mammals and much longer for fish, amphibians etc. You should therefore decapitate an animal only when it is *un*conscious: stun it first if necessary. Decapitation after stunning is often used on amphibians, reptiles and fish like eels, sharks and rays.

Asphyxiation

This is the prevention of breathing by pressure on the windpipe or by blocking off the animal's air intake. It should never be used as a method of humane killing except in an emergency, and then only if the animal is already unconscious. Depending on the animal's size, put either your foot (for dog or fox) or a stick or pencil across the windpipe and press hard. Drowning is another form of asphyxiation but do not use it. Over the years innumerable kittens and puppies have suffered horribly by this "kind" method of killing unwanted litters.

Exsanguination (Bleeding or Throat-slitting)

To ensure that an animal really is dead—and only use this method if it is already unconscious—cut the major blood vessels, that is, the carotid arteries and jugular veins and let the blood gush out.

Cardiac Arrest

A simple method for **bats, small birds** and other **small creatures** with delicate bones. Squeeze the ribcage firmly between thumb and finger to stop the breathing and the heartbeat. A bird should be on its back so that you can press its sternum firmly to compress the heart and lungs: it will instantly become unconscious and will die soon afterwards.

Chilling and Heating

Tropical **fish** and tropical **crustaceans** will die if cooled to 4 °C or below, and cold-water fish and crustaceans will die below freezing point but will suffer if this is done slowly. Put them straight into a deepfreeze at −20 °C so that they freeze to death rapidly. The same method can be used for **invertebrates.**

Overheating also kills: for example, mammals die if their body temperature exceeds 45 °C. However, the only semi-humane method of killing by overheating is the boiling of crustaceans and invertebrates. It is not nice. Smaller crustaceans like shrimps take only a few seconds to die in fast-boiling salt water but lobsters and crabs take at least 15 seconds and object violently to the whole business.

Chemical Euthanasia

The main chemical methods are by gas inhalation or by an overdose of injected anaesthetics (the animal is quite literally "put to sleep"). These methods can only be used under veterinary supervision and instruction.

Disposal

Whoever has given the animal its release from suffering is generally responsible for disposing of its body, either by burying, or by burning, or in sealed black plastic sacks to the local public tip or incinerator. However, if the animal was diseased or its body contains residual drugs so that it might be dangerous to other (scavenging) animals or people, you should seek advice on disposal from the police, a veterinary surgeon or your local authority's environmental health department.

The bodies of badgers (whether found dead of natural causes or given mercy killing) should be offered to the Ministry of Agriculture, Fisheries and Food (MAFF; DAFS in Scotland) for autopsy because of the possible link with bovine tuberculosis. Bob Stebbings at the Institute of Terrestrial Ecology is always grateful for the bodies of dead bats: either contact the NCC or your local bat group, or pack the body in plenty of tissue in a polythene bag within a stout cardboard box and post it immediately to Dr Stebbings with a note of where it was found and under what circumstances.

The disposal of the bodies of whales, porpoises and dolphins is the responsibility of the county council (cetaceans are "royal fish" and are the property of the Crown in coastal waters), but the district council is responsible for collecting the carcase.

CHAPTER SIX

EMERGENCY ACCOMMODATION

There are many factors you need to take into account when considering suitable accommodation for an animal, but keep your ideas as simple as possible. Think animal: consider the habits of the species, the age and sex of the animal, its problem and general condition, and aim to provide it with security and comfort so that it can rest. Think ahead: try and provide accommodation which will be adequate, or can easily be made so, for each stage of the animal's recovery while you are its host, because it will need a familiar base "nest" or den throughout that period—try and let it have the same base within whatever larger space it is eventually confined. Keep it basically simple, but the longer the patient's stay, the more need it will have for environmental stimulation.

Whatever kind of accommodation you offer, whether humble or purpose-built, it is essential that it should be scrupulously clean before a new patient is put into it. One of the advantages of makeshift containers like cardboard boxes is that they are disposable and are burned after use, so that there is little risk of a lingering infection or a build-up of fungi, bacteria, parasites and other pathogens lying in wait to attack an animal already weakened by the circumstances of its distress.

Finally, but most importantly, think about **water.** All the vital information and advice on this subject has been gathered at the end of this chapter and should not be overlooked.

BIRDS

The first need of a shocked bird (and that includes virtually any wild bird which has been handled or confined) is somewhere warm, dark and quiet. Quite often that is all the care it will need, and very often the lack of such a place to regain its composure will either kill a bird which would otherwise have survived or greatly prolong its need for care.

Cardboard boxes are ideal if they are dry, clean and airy. A distressed bird should not be able to see out of its container, nor feel that it is being watched, and for these reasons it will not be at all happy in a typical draughty budgie or parrot cage, which might be your first idea, but if that is all you have to hand, cover it with a dark cloth (without suffocating the bird!) and put it in a warm room where there will be no disturbance. A bird of prey is best left in its travelling container, certainly for the first night as long as there is enough space for it to stand without being cramped. Any distressed bird needs an ambient temperature of at least 25 °C—preferably 26 °C. An airing cupboard is fine for a while for a small or very young bird in a box: it is warm and dark and, unless you have a noisy plumbing system, reasonably peaceful.

If you happen to have an incubator or a brooder, scrub it out and use it, or consider an aquarium or a plant propagator with a built-in heating system, or a purpose-built heated hospital cage (solid-sided except for the front) from an avicultural supplier (see Fig. 36 on p. 128). However, beware of overheating. A dull-emitter infra-red lamp, like those used for brooding chicks or young farm animals, is a good source of heat if you have one as is a hot-water bottle, well wrapped up and padded. Light bulbs are another source of heat but should be red at this stage as the bird needs subdued light or darkness for at least the first few hours. To retain the heat, insulate the container with an outer layer of, say, foam or polystyrene, as long as there is absolutely no risk of the material catching fire.

After the initial recovery period of intensive care in dark and warmth, the bird will need more space and can be given a little more light, though still subdued. It still needs lack of disturbance and must be able to hide from prying eyes if it wishes. Even human patients appreciate privacy and a wild creature much more so, especially a bird, for whom out of sight is out of mind.

The new accommodation should allow at least enough space for the bird to stretch its wings, preen itself and preferably move about with a reasonable degree of freedom: it is not a battery hen. But the space should still restrict the bird so that it cannot injure itself by flapping around.

Many birds are social within their species and are also used to mixing with other species, so that it can be reassuring for them to be able to see other birds once they are over the first few hours of darkness, warmth and privacy. But be careful with territorial types, who will do their best to get at each other in spite of their cages—and certainly do *not* have a predator bird in sight of other species: it will terrify them just with its eyes and shape.

Give some thought to the level at which a bird is housed. Waterfowl and landfowl are happy enough at ground level but most birds live most of their lives off the ground—in flight, perching in shrubs or trees, or on cliffs perhaps—and are not used to being confined somewhere at or below human eye-level. Try and put them as high as possible in the room if they are caged.

The base of the accommodation needs bedding for warmth and to absorb droppings but do not use hay, straw or similar dry and dusty materials which might lead to respiratory infection. Use thick layers of newspaper, paper towels, or clean old cloths, but avoid towelling in case its loops catch claws. If you use cloths, make sure that every trace of detergent has been rinsed out of them because it can adversely affect a bird's plumage, especially in the case of waterfowl and seabirds. Be a little careful with newspaper: it can make rather a slippery surface for some birds and after a while some species could develop splayed legs, especially if they are growing youngsters. In some cases, a more suitable floor covering is sods or moist peat and sand.

Perching birds naturally appreciate a perch if they are not suffering from leg injuries. Use natural materials (branches etc., but avoid yew and most other conifers).

Birds of prey will do well at this stage in something like a tea-chest or big wooden crate with enough space to spread their wings (which can be of a considerable span) and a fairly thick perch which does not let their talons curve into the balls of their feet. The box will need disposable coverings on the inside of its back wall as well as on the floor, to absorb the somewhat explosive and more or less horizontal ejection of droppings by many diurnal raptors.

Large fowl like peacocks need broad, flat perches (perhaps a piece of 4 inch by 2 inch timber) and a lot more space to accommodate their long tails without damaging them. Other pheasants (yes, peafowl are pheasants—so are chickens) and gamebirds will be quieter in darkened accommodation as usual, and like to hide at ground level if they think they are being observed. Many of them need to remain quite closely confined or they will damage themselves in persistent and sometimes frantic efforts to escape, especially if there are people in sight. Alternatively, give them a lot of space and absolute privacy with the freedom of a warm room (but not on a slippery floor surface), leaving food and water available and keeping out of sight as much as possible. Offer the bird somewhere to hide when you enter the room—perhaps a few conifer branches in a corner. It will be much happier in an outdoor pen as soon as it is able to do without extra warmth.

Quail are best kept in close confinement with a padded ceiling low enough to remind them it is there. If they are put in an aviary at some stage, give it a false ceiling of soft string mesh or hessian sacking to soften the impact when they rocket skywards in a panic.

Waders (including herons, coots, moorhens and other birds with long legs for paddling but unwebbed feet) are much happier outside than in but will need to be kept inside at first, preferably loose in a private room. Like gamebirds, they too need somewhere to hide but it can be a very simple screen. The floor needs something like sawdust rather than slippery newspaper, but make sure the sawdust has no trace of preservatives or other chemicals in it. Like oiled seabirds, waders as a group need at least twenty-four hours of absolute peace and privacy after capture.

Seabirds can either be closely confined in a typical hospital cage, preferably with another of their own species and size for company, or can be given the freedom of a concrete-floored room well padded with newspaper. However, if several of them are loose together, they tend to panic when someone enters the room and are therefore better in cages initially.

Swans, geese and ducks—some ducks, such as mallard or their domesticated relations, are fairly easy to house, the biggest problem being their copious liquid droppings and their need to dunk their food in water which causes the whole area to become soaking wet. Their short-term intensive care quarters can be the standard cardboard box with plenty of newspaper in the base but they will need something bigger and more easily managed very soon. Some people put them in a sink or bath (*without* bathing water). A low chicken run would be invaluable for ducks, especially the type attached to its own coop or ark.

All the wildfowl are quite happy without any housing out of doors; rain does not bother them and is in fact essential for their plumage if they have no swimming pond, as long as it is a shower rather than a downpour. However, they do appreciate wind-breaks—perhaps straw bales here and there or shrubbery or weather boards. If birds are penned out of doors in small enclosures like chicken arks (which have the virtue of being portable so that you can give fresh ground at intervals), have the sense not to put them on an exposed site. All the wildfowl do better on grass than permanently on concrete, which could produce sore, dry feet, but the grass will not remain grass for long unless the pen can be shifted regularly.

Geese and swans are large birds, and a fully grown swan could have a wingspan of as much as 7 feet across. If a wing is damaged, space should be restricted to deter it from flapping, but otherwise any bird needs to be able to have a good stretch and a feather-settling flap now and then, so there should be adequate space to avoid the wings being injured against the sides of the accommodation. Whereas a wild duck needs a ceiling of some kind to prevent it from flying off before its time, swans are quite incapable of taking off without several yards of runway, preferably on water (they need even more space on land) and therefore overhead wire-netting is not necessary. However, if wildfowl want to fly off, they are possibly fit to do so and should not be prevented unless conditions dictate otherwise.

Access to sunshine in moderation is an important aid to recuperation and some swans and geese have been very content in a well-windowed barn or garden shed, or even in a greenhouse, though that is like being in a goldfish bowl, and a solar-heated one at that. If a greenhouse is the only possible accommodation, give it adequate ventilation and watch the temperature carefully. Make sure that the glass is thoroughly dirty outside (spray it with whitewash if necessary) so that the bird knows the glass is there, and so that the sun's heat is deflected. Also put some kind of temporary cladding rising perhaps 2 or 3 feet from ground level for privacy: no bird, however big, will appreciate seeing a dog, cat or nocturnal fox peering through the glass at it.

MAMMALS

Like birds, the immediate needs of distressed mammals are privacy, peace, darkness and warmth—but not necessarily artificial heating, as long as they can snuggle into warm bedding and are free from draughts and chill.

For the first few hours at least, wild mammals other than deer should be allowed to remain in their travelling containers, which will have become familiar to them and give some sense of security. The container can be placed somewhere undisturbed and, although you can put it in a larger confined area to which the animal has free access, it is more than likely to remain hidden in its "den" or "nest" for preference while it recovers. The accommodation described below for different species is for emergency use only; more appropriate housing for the recuperation phases is described in the Rehabilitation chapter.

Deer

Deer are much more difficult to accommodate at all stages than other mammals, wild or domesticated. They, too, need peace, darkness and adequate warmth while they are in a state of shock but indoor confinement could cause considerable stress, even if it does not show. Give them a good paddock with plenty of natural bushy cover in which they can feel safe, or provide some random screens of straw bales or wattle hurdles. An incapacitated deer will need overhead protection from heavy rain: in summer a leafy tree will do the job but otherwise you will need to provide an artificial arrangement which avoids giving any sense of confinement. On a farm, an open pole barn would be ideal, and indeed several wildlife veterinary practices have a good network of local farmers willing to accommodate injured deer.

Badgers, Foxes and Otters

Foxes and badgers will have a strong urge to go to ground in a dark, secret place. A dog kennel could serve the purpose, or put the travelling container in a shed or unused garage, placing it so that daylight does not fall on the container's entrance every time you open the shed door. Try something like a tea-chest at the back of the shed in one corner, set with its opening facing the side wall so that the gap between the opening and the wall is just big enough for the animal to use as an entrance (see Fig. 43 on p. 183). Give plenty of bedding hay or straw but no artificial heating. If there is a risk of draughts at floor level, raise the den a few inches on a platform—perhaps an old pallet or some timbers—which will also lift the den out of the way of chill and damp rising from a solid floor. A large and thoroughly scrubbed out dustbin on its side, staunchly wedged so that it cannot roll, could provide a good den within an enclosure, or for emergency overnight confinement use an upright dustbin with a lid and airholes and ample bedding in the base so that the animal can curl up and rest. Put plenty of sawdust on the shed floor to absorb urine and to give further insulation.

A tea-chest could also be used for an otter, as long as it is within a room or shed. As you would for a badger or fox, put the "den" in a quiet corner facing sideways with just enough of a gap for the animal to get in and out. Watch out for hazards like electrical fittings in the room.

Unless they are very sick indeed, badgers will probably resent being confined and are powerful enough to claw their way out of most situations, including wooden sheds—and could be frantic enough to lacerate their feet by scrabbling furiously at concrete. Some foxes are also determined escapologists (they can climb as well as dig and chew) but others seem to accept the situation quite amicably. In the longer term (more than a night or two) it is far better for these larger wild mammals to be housed by someone who already has proper accommodation and expertise, unless you are prepared to go to considerable lengths, and expense, to build something appropriate quickly. In the meantime, it is wiser not to be tempted to keep a fox in the house: its musk can be potent, pervasive and persistent.

Rodents and Insectivores

Smaller wild mammals are much easier, though active species like squirrels, mustelids, lagomorphs (rabbits and hares) and rats can be a handful and a headache. Most of the rest can be kept easily enough in, say, a converted aquarium with a lid, a hamster cage, a hospital cage, a large cake tin with airholes in the lid—in fact, anything which cannot be chewed or dug through or jumped or climbed out of. Do not make airholes too big: some **mice,** for example, can squeeze through any hole big enough to get your thumb into and indeed some would say any hole big enough to take a ballpoint pen. For these smaller creatures, punch airholes with a nail, but do something about the jagged edges.

Within the container, give the animal a nest of sweet hay, preferably tucked into an inner box for privacy and warmth. A **mole** would prefer a layer of soil deep enough for it to burrow into instead. **Hedgehogs** are usually peaceful patients and not exactly athletic (though they can be good climbers) and can be kept in the first instance in a cardboard box with ample bedding like dry dead leaves, hay or straw. If the room is hazard free, let the hedgehog potter out of its box when it wants, which will probably be at night, but once it begins to feel better it will be an active climber and needs a better enclosure (see Rehabilitation chapter).

Bats do best in small wooden cages. Provide a very rough surface or line the inside of the wood (including the ceiling) with wire mesh so that the bat can hang upside down in its customary manner (see Fig. 37). Think of bats in the attic and devise something appropriate: imagine them clinging with the claws of their back feet among the rafters and in cavity walls. They need enough room to be able to stretch out one wing at a time when grooming. Give them seclusion, and at first give them artificial heat; at 25–30 °C they keep active, and that seems to speed recovery. It could even be as high as 34–36 °C in the intensive care period and an airing cupboard is an ideal environment in the short term, as long as there is adequate humidity.

Squirrels, Lagomorphs and Small Mustelids

These more active species need larger and more cunningly escape-proof accommodation, even when quite ill. All the rodents can gnaw their way to freedom, especially **squirrels,** which deeply resent confinement and are almost claustrophobic. A squirrel would probably be best in a metal cage: the metal will defy its teeth (though it will still try) and the openness of a cage will make it feel less claustrophobic; a cloth can be draped over part of the cage to give it seclusion. Put sawdust on the floor and provide nesting material.

All the **mustelids** (like stoats, weasels and ferrets) are superb escapologists; they climb, they dig, and they can slip through remarkably small chinks. There are many designs of ferret cage which could also be used for their wild relatives, and in principle they have three definite areas: dining room, living room with bathroom, and bedroom. They do need an inner sanctuary which is warm, dark and completely private, with a smallish entry hole and of hay inside: they like to bury themselves completely in a good warm bed and will disappear from view in a curled-up ball (see Fig. 38).

FIG. 36 HOSPITAL CAGE FOR BIRDS

Good ventilation, humidity control, artificial heating and temperature control are vital. This simple example has a dull-emitter infra-red lamp attached to the cage front. (Also suitable for small mammals.)

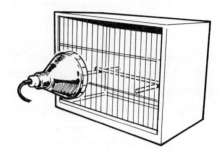

FIG. 37 HOSPITAL CAGE FOR BATS

Mesh on inside walls and ceiling makes good clinging surface for roosting.

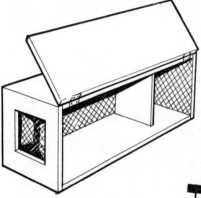

FIG. 38 STANDARD FERRET HUTCH

Suitable for other small mustelids but mesh must be rigid, strong and of appropriately small diameter. Metal reinforcement probably required for wild mustelids.

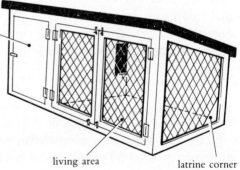

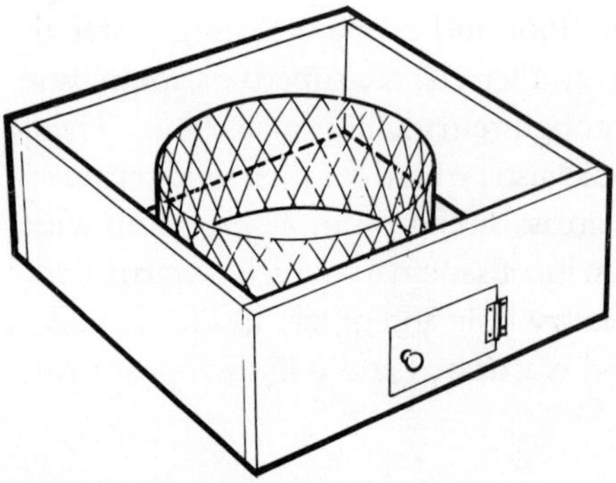

"bedroom"

living area

latrine corner

FIG. 39 HAYBOX BROODER FOR CHICKS

Basic frame is wooden or hardboard box, containing circular wire-mesh pen for the chicks. Fill space between box and pen with hay to retain warmth.

A good rabbit hutch, like a good ferret hutch, also provides three defined areas—bedroom, dining room and bathroom. **Rabbits and hares** find capture extremely traumatic and for the first night they should be left in complete privacy, peace and darkness, with ample bedding, water and some greenstuff. Do not even think of examining, handling or treating them until the following day. They are much less adept at escaping, though they will try digging, and you can probably improvise emergency accommodation with a tea-chest and some chicken wire.

Domestic Mammals

Domestic mammals are much simpler to accommodate: they are used to humans and are not usually desperate to escape. **Dogs and cats** need somewhere warm and undisturbed, with an emergency open cardboard box for a bed well supplied with clean old blankets and protected from floor draughts. Leave them in a quiet, dark room in privacy and put plenty of newspaper on the floor as well as providing a litter-tray for a cat. Other pets like **hamsters** and **tame mice** can be put in hospital cages, empty aquariums, or pet cages with three solid sides to keep them warm and a good supply of bedding hay or straw in the corner at the back where they can hide themselves. Sick adult **goats and sheep** need a warm, dry shed but also good ventilation without draughts: they need a dry bed on soft, clean, bright straw with no hint of mustiness. Sick **cattle, donkeys and horses** need indoor accommodation, preferably in a loose-box, and might need rugging. All livestock need immediate and constant access to a generous supply of fresh drinking water at all times.

Marine Mammals

Do not even try to accommodate a marine mammal: it is essential that they have expert attention in proper surroundings. Warning has already been given not to pick up baby seals from the beach but people persist in doing so and then take them home and put them in the bath, risking the life of what was probably a perfectly healthy, happy animal.

AMPHIBIANS, REPTILES AND INSECTS

Amphibians and reptiles need peace and minimal handling. Initially they can be kept in a well-ventilated, lidded box with sand or newspaper on the floor. Amphibians need access to shallow bathing water and a damp atmosphere: reptilian requirements vary according to species (see Rehabilitation chapter).

A simple aquarium can also be used for many kinds of insect, or you could use a terrarium or, of course, a ventilated matchbox in the short term.

WATER

Water is life to all creatures and fresh, clean drinking water should be available at all times, whatever the species. Many casualties will need water as a priority and will often have to be encouraged to drink. Fluid replacement is a vital part of treatment for shock and is often given in the form of a glucose-saline solution by injection.

With some creatures, drinking water is an immediate necessity. For example, **bats** must be given water as soon as possible, and certainly before they are fed: use an eye-dropper or a syringe to dribble water into their mouths. Use the same equipment for **birds** and give them warm water with glucose dissolved in it. A small bird needs a few drops squeezed in at the hinge of its beak at two-hourly intervals during daylight hours until it is able to drink of its own accord (the glucose gives immediate sustenance) and a bird as big as a crow needs perhaps half a teaspoonful at similar intervals. Be very careful not to choke the bird: be gentle and drip the water into the mouth slowly and carefully, giving the bird plenty of time to swallow. If a bird is eating, or is being force-fed, you can dip alternate pieces of its food into water, shaking off the excess, to make sure that it does get moisture. Some birds get most of their liquid intake in their natural food: the bodies of juicy caterpillars, for example.

Birds need water for several purposes, primarily for drinking and for bathing in. Some also need it for dunking their food; some can only defecate in water; some find safety from predators by resting on the water; some use water to make mud for building their nests. It is important to cater for all these requirements separately in a confined and unnatural situation, unless you can provide a constant through-flow of water in a self-cleaning system. Apart from the restrictions on oiled birds discussed in Chapter 4, all birds should be offered the opportunity to bathe, even if they refuse it—in which case it might be beneficial to spray them with a fine mist of water now and then if they have no access to rain showers. Unless there are good veterinary reasons against it, hospitalised birds can be mist-sprayed or given a shallow bathing bowl—just half an inch for small birds, and only an inch for a bigger bird like an owl. Waterfowl and seabirds will suffer if their feet do not have regular access to water, and many diving and dabbling birds need to be able to get their heads under water at intervals in order to keep their eyes and nostrils in good condition. Bathing not only cleans feathers and removes parasites but it also encourages a bird to preen, which is essential to keeping its plumage in good condition.

This only applies to adults: chicks and hand-reared ducklings, for example, should not be allowed to bathe. Bathing water for patients should be at about 40 °C and should be kept quite separate from drinking water, which is best put in a small container (not big enough to bathe in) above ground level and at a natural temperature—cooler rather than warmer in most circumstances. Many birds reject water which has been warmed by the sun but are quite happy to drink it icy cold. In winter in an outdoor aviary, however, drinking water needs to be kept free of ice: use a metal dish and put it on bricks with a night-light underneath or on a tile pipe which houses a light bulb, or use a thermostatically controlled immersion heater, or devise a constant circulation system to prevent ice formation, perhaps by means of a submersible pump or fountain of the type used in garden pools and aquariums.

Above all, drinking water must always be absolutely clean and fresh. Some birds seem to drink very little, especially those who find moisture in their food, but even so they should be given every opportunity to drink whenever they wish. The drier the diet, the greater the need.

Wild birds might not at first recognise drinking water in an artificial container, and it is standard practice for gamekeepers and poultry rearers to dip the beaks of new chicks in the water to give them the right idea when they are first introduced into new quarters. A dish of water can be more attractive if the water "moves": try rippling its surface with the occasional drip. Chicks and older fowl are usually given water from drinkers specifically designed to avoid contamination of the water by faeces, food and floor litter.

All **mammals** also need constant access to fresh, clean drinking water and you need to give some thought to water containers. Foxes, for example, tend to urinate in their water; other animals do their best to tip over a water bowl. Mammals like rabbits, ferrets and cage pets can be taught to use drinking bottles: a plastic bottleful of water is hooked on the outside of the cage, with a plastic drinking tube projecting into the cage, so that the source remains uncontaminated. If a container is put in an animal's accommodation, make sure it is untippable and place it well away from any customary defecation area (many animals are very specific in their latrine habits). Consider raising the vessel above ground level but still low enough for a natural drinking attitude. Hedgehogs, incidentally, drink a great deal for their size—Les Stocker suggests up to a fifth of a pint at a time.

Large mammals like horses and especially cattle drink substantial amounts of water: a cow in milk, for example, can get through many gallons a day. They need a constant *running* supply such as that provided by a ballcock tank off the mains, unless you are prepared to use a hose for regular top-ups during the day. Sheep and goats are much less thirsty but still need access to clean, fresh water, especially if they are eating hay rather than grass (which in spring has a high moisture content).

Amphibians and reptiles also need constant access to water, whether for drinking or for swimming. Snakes do need to drink, and adders are especially thirsty. Amphibians must be able to immerse themselves in water, especially in the breeding season, and frogs sometimes hibernate at the bottom of a pond in winter.

CHAPTER SEVEN

FEEDING

In most cases, food is not an immediate requirement for a distressed animal: peace, warmth, rest and water are more important. However, suitable food should be made freely available and occasionally a patient will need force-feeding, or at least encouragement to eat. A problem with wild creatures is that they might not recognise what is offered as being edible, especially if they are used to catching live food in their natural environment, but there are various tricks you can try to persuade them to eat. Force-feeding should be a last resort.

Before you can offer food, it is essential to identify the species so that you can devise a diet which is at least approximately appropriate. Ideally, of course, you would scour the countryside for the animal's natural food but in fact nearly every species can survive, and even thrive, on foods you are likely to find in your own larder or at the local pet-shop or agricultural feed merchant. A word of warning: many people use bread and milk as emergency food, and even as a staple diet, but this could be unsuitable and even harmful for many species.

The most useful standby foods you can have in your kitchen for any creature, wild or domesticated (apart from large herbivores), include the following:

Water!
Glucose
Eggs
Cheddar cheese and cottage
  cheese
Complan, Farex and other
  infant/invalid foods
Unsalted peanuts
Sunflower seeds
Ox liver or heart or fresh
  minced beef

Tins of dog or cat food
Puppy meal
Wholemeal bread
Peanut butter
Frozen sprats
Tinned pilchards
Assorted fruit and nuts
Honey
Green vegetables

If you are likely to have more than the occasional animal casualty on your hands, you should also stock:

Sluis Universal or some other insectivorous food
Lamlac ewe-milk replacer for orphans
Frozen goat's milk and colostrum
Lectade oral rehydration fluid
Mazuri Zoo Food A
Veterinary oral multi-vitamin supplement (e.g. Abidec, Vionate)
Frozen day-old chicks and laboratory "pinkies"
Gizzard grit and calcium (e.g. crushed oyster-shell, snail-shells or egg-shells; cuttlefish)
Grain and poultry pellets
Live invertebrate breeding colonies (e.g. mealworms, grasshoppers, wax-moths, fruit flies, earthworms)
Hydroponic grasses
Growing garden weeds and comfrey

ENCOURAGEMENT AND FORCE-FEEDING

Any creature unwilling to feed is probably in serious trouble, either because it is close to death, or because of internal injuries or because it is mechanically unable to eat as a result of, say, a broken jaw or bill or an obstruction in the throat. Sometimes, however, apparent lack of appetite is due to the shock of capture and confinement (adders rarely feed in captivity) or an inability to recognise what it is offered as food. For example, raptors and carnivorous mammals are used to catching live food and, unless they habitually eat carrion, they will probably reject dead offerings or inanimate lumps of raw meat and dogfood. Seabirds often find difficulty in recognising dead fish, and the same is true for kingfishers.

The way in which food is presented is as important as finding appropriate food in the first place, and you need to find out as much as possible about the creature's natural habits. Some birds only feed on the ground while others feel safer perching above it; many waterfowl will only take food presented in or on water, or need to be able to dunk the food themselves; some birds, especially swallows, swifts and flycatchers, feed only while on the wing. Some small insectivorous mammals need to eat almost constantly just to stay alive, while larger carnivores are used to gorging while they can and going without for perhaps a day or two when hunting is poor. The time of year is another factor: hibernating or semi-hibernating creatures need to accumulate fat before winter and thereafter eat rarely; many birds adjust their diet according to what is available seasonally; many amphibians and fish and several birds are carnivorous at one stage of their lives but largely vegetarian or omnivorous at others. You should also take the time of day into account: does the animal normally feed in daylight, or is it a dusk diner like a badger or a nocturnal hunter like an owl? Adjust your own routines to suit the animal's diurnal/nocturnal rhythms.

The species notes in Appendix 3 give some guidance on natural diets and eating habits, with hints on standby foods and feeding methods, and you should try every trick to let an animal feed itself within a reasonable period. Only force-feed if it is essential to do so, because the very act of force-feeding is traumatic (for you as well as for the animal) and also requires both patience and expertise. Quite often all you need to do is to give the animal a taste of the food—for example, smear a bat's lips with the juicy innards of a mealworm—or get a similar domesticated species to set an example (a canary could show wild finches that a seed dish is a source of food). Try hiding food in places where an inquisitive creature would expect to look for it—in the crevices of a piece of bark for birds like nuthatches, say—or catch the eye of an insectivorous bird or mammal by putting something live and wiggly on a bowl of food, like a mealworm or two. Remember that wild creatures will probably be very suspicious of a food dish, though some (like hedgehogs) will treat it like a stone and tip it over to see what is underneath.

Emergency Measures

If there is an urgent need to counteract either dehydration or starvation, a veterinary surgeon will probably give a subcutaneous injection of a glucose-saline solution with vitamins and probably an oral dose of electrolyte replacer to restore the balance of certain metabolically essential cellular salts. Restoration of those balances is essentially a veterinary procedure but your vet will be able to teach you how to administer the replacer fluids. In an emergency, make up a drink of glucose dissolved in warm water (a tablespoonful of glucose to a pint of water) and give it by mouth if the animal is conscious, at a rate of say 5 per cent of the patient's bodyweight daily in two or three doses. Do not use sugar instead of glucose.

Glucose or dextrose solutions not only help with restoring the body fluid balance but also begin to supply metabolisable energy to keep an animal alive. If there is no suitable food available in an emergency, give a 10 per cent solution of glucose in warm water by mouth at a rate of 10 ml/kg bodyweight at half-hourly intervals, supplemented with something like a lamb tonic, until something more substantial can be given by subcutaneous injection by a vet (for example, Duphalyte includes amino acids and vitamins).

These are emergency life-saving measures which in most cases you would ask a vet to handle. In less drastic situations, you might need to force-feed at home, especially in the case of a starving bird. Injured birds might not have been able to find food for some time, but in some cases you will do more harm than good by trying to force-feed them, especially if the bird has a long, fragile beak. In other cases force-feeding should be left to the experts, either because amateur attempts will endanger the animal or because it could be dangerous for the handler. Make sure that you do offer appropriate food: if an animal is left to help itself to food, it can reject the unsuitable, but if it is force-fed it has no choice in the matter.

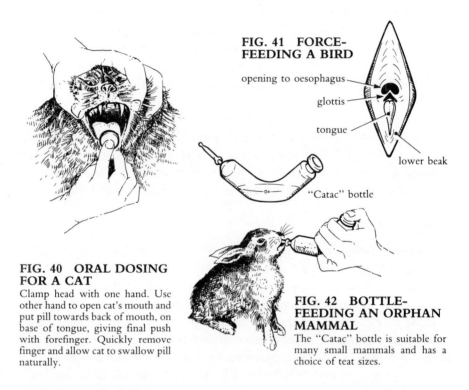

FIG. 41   FORCE-FEEDING A BIRD

opening to oesophagus

glottis

tongue

lower beak

"Catac" bottle

FIG. 40   ORAL DOSING FOR A CAT
Clamp head with one hand. Use other hand to open cat's mouth and put pill towards back of mouth, on base of tongue, giving final push with forefinger. Quickly remove finger and allow cat to swallow pill naturally.

FIG. 42   BOTTLE-FEEDING AN ORPHAN MAMMAL
The "Catac" bottle is suitable for many small mammals and has a choice of teat sizes.

Force-feeding Birds

The aim is to get suitable food into the bird's stomach by way of its mouth. That means you need to be able to open the beak and to pass the food into its oesophagus or gullet (which leads into the crop and the digestive tract) rather than into the trachea or windpipe (which leads into the respiratory system). It is vital that you choose the right path, or the animal will choke or drown (see Fig. 41). The signpost is the glottis, which is the opening to the windpipe: you can see it at the back of the tongue where it opens and closes in time with the bird's breathing. The glottis closes during swallowing, in order to protect the lungs. If you need to use a stomach tube for force-feeding, you must ensure that it is not pushed through the glottis in error; you should also take care to avoid the glottis if you are pushing food in with your fingers or a pair of blunt forceps. The proper opening to the gullet is beyond the glottis and is much bigger.

To open a bird's beak, concentrate on the hinge: never try and force open the tips. If you only want to trickle liquids into the back of the mouth so that the bird can be encouraged to swallow them, use a matchstick or toothpick on a small bird and insert it firmly but gently between the upper and lower halves of the beak near the hinge to prise them apart. Some birds, especially wildfowl, will be persuaded to open up if you apply gentle pressure at the hinge. Seabirds tend to have strong jaw muscles and it can be a bit of a struggle to open their beaks. With birds of prey, it should be fairly easy to raise the *upper* beak, and that will automatically depress the lower half—but do not force them too wide apart. For all these larger birds, two people are needed: one to hold the bird while the other opens the beak and does the feeding. The holder should ensure that strong-billed birds are not able to stab at the feeder: the bird should be held firmly just behind its head until the feeder has control of its beak. With birds of prey, make sure that their talons are firmly embedded in a cushion or something, with their bodyweight pressing down on it so that they cannot strike out. You can often encourage some birds of prey to take a piece of meat from blunted forceps by touching the sensitive gape-feathers at the corner of the mouth, but watch out for the grab they will make at the food.

Never try and force open the beak of a wader. Most of them are anyway very nervous, and force-feeding will cause them to vomit, which nullifies the effect of the food. Long beaks are particularly vulnerable and if you really must insert a stomach tube you need to take great care in opening the beak or you will damage it. Slip something as thin as a thumbnail between the two halves near the hinge and part them very gently. Do everything slowly and kindly to try and mitigate the bird's distress.

In many cases, force-feeding is only a matter of placing a **pellet** of food at the back of the tongue and encouraging the bird to swallow it. This method can also be used to give medicines disguised in food. Open the beak and use your fingers to put the pellet of food to the back of the throat, beyond the glottis, then push it carefully down the gullet with your finger or with a pair of blunted forceps (wrap tape round the tips).

Invalid foods like Complan, Farex, Build-up, Farlene, or Pedigree Petfood's convalescent diet—designed for cats and dogs but suitable for most birds—can be made up to a suitable texture so that they can be put in a plastic **syringe** (chop off the syringe's nozzle to make a bigger hole) and then either extruded to look like little worms, which the bird will probably pick up of its own accord, or squeezed out in blobs at the back of the throat well beyond the glottis (this idea comes from the Liverpool veterinary surgeon and author, Brian Coles).

An **oesophagal or stomach tube** takes the food past the swallowing stage, if that has proved difficult or undesirable. Gently open the bird's beak, as already described, and have its head and neck extended more or less vertically so that there is a fairly direct line down the throat to the crop. Use a rubber tube of a diameter and length appropriate to the size of bird, boiled beforehand to make sure it is absolutely sterile and then given a lubricating coat of liquid paraffin to ease its passage down the bird's gullet. Push it very gently down the oesophagus, avoiding the glottis. Do not force it down: the bird is already under enough stress as it is, though because of the relatively large size of a bird's gullet it is easier than trying to give a mammal a stomach tube. Do make sure that the tube does not disappear completely down the poor bird's throat: keep a firm hold on the free end in case the whole thing gets swallowed.

With the tube in place, fill a syringe with an appropriate food of a consistency that will pass easily down the tube. (Liquids can be trickled carefully into a funnel at the top of the tube, with no need for a syringe unless you want to measure the bird's intake.) Push the stuff down the tube gradually, gently but steadily. If it comes back up, you need to slow down the rate. Use a food which can be quickly assimilated so that the bird's digestive system has less work to make the food available to its body. Either ask your vet to supply something appropriate or use human invalid foods like Complan or even tinned baby food. In general terms, a healthy, active small bird in the wild would eat the equivalent of up to a third of its own bodyweight a day, and a bigger bird up to a seventh (the bigger the bird, the smaller the ratio of its body surface to body volume and therefore the lower its rate of heat loss).

Wildfowl usually eat very readily: if they have not eaten for two days and have no obvious obstruction, use a stomach tube to give them a thickish mix of either fish purée or baby cereal, depending on their normal diet.

Seabirds should not be force-fed for at least twenty-four hours. If feeding is necessary, give them whole fish, head first, by opening the bird's beak and pushing the fish well down into its throat. Choose a size of fish the bird can swallow easily (sprats for most, perhaps mackerel for a gannet) and give it two fish twice a day, leaving a help-yourself supply for the rest of the time. The moment it does begin to help itself, stop force-feeding. That applies to all force-feeding: it should be stopped at the earliest possible moment.

Raptors will usually take food, once they realise what it is, and you will probably have to offer strips of raw meat at first with the aid of blunted forceps. Dip the meat in water to moisten it, and the same applies if you are offering them dead day-old hatchery chicks. Open the bird's beak, pop the food at the back of the tongue, close the beak and stroke the throat to encourage swallowing: you should be able to see or feel the act of swallowing. Use a regime of six days on, one off: for example, a kestrel can be given one chick the first, third and fifth days, two chicks the second, fourth and sixth days and none at all on the seventh.

Waders should not really be force-fed at all, for reasons already explained, but if it is essential you should adminster food by stomach tube, very slowly, and then leave the bird alone as soon as the job is done. **Gamebirds** are as nervous as waders and are not candidates for force-feeding: if they won't eat, then they have a very serious and probably irreparable problem. They are natural tit-bitters who feed by pecking at anything which might be edible and so they should have little hesitation in picking up food morsels from the ground.

Most **other species** of bird should not be force-fed except as a last resort, when they can be given pellets of, say, finely grated hard-boiled egg mixed with dampened breadcrumbs, or pieces of scrambled egg, put right at the back of the tongue and perhaps helped down with a drop or two of water. However, the exception are **swifts,** who very often will not feed themselves in captivity and who are quite easy to force-feed because they do not seem to be too worried by their proximity to people and they will gape very wide to be helpful!

Force-feeding Wild Mammals

Mammals are much more difficult to force-feed than birds, and the general rule is—don't. Try everything you can think of to tempt the animal to eat; offer it soft foods or even soups and purée if it has an injury that makes the mechanics of eating difficult. Be ingenious in your choice and presentation of food, and remember that carnivores are quite used to occasional fasting in the absence of prey, though some of the insectivores, especially shrews and moles, do need to eat frequently, that is every few hours, in order to survive.

One mammal worth trying to force-feed is, surprisingly, a **deer.** If it will not feed itself, its chances of recovery are slim but you could try feeding it by squeezing and dribbling something like Lactol, Complan or baby cereal into the side of its mouth with a syringe or a clean squeezy bottle. Make up the food as thick as possible, and be very, very patient, feeding it gently and carefully. One of the larger species would need perhaps a pint two or three times a day. A similar method can be used for a **hedgehog** which cannot feed itself: trickle a warm glucose solution into the corner of the mouth with the help of a syringe.

The standard way of force-feeding **farm livestock** like cattle, sheep and goats is to give them a "drench", which is not as drastic as it sounds and is fairly similar to the method of feeding a deer just described. Drenching is used regularly on the farm to give medicines, rehydrants, and liquid nourishment, and a farmer or a vet will be able to demonstrate the technique.

FEEDING BIRDS

If a bird *will* eat, and can eat, what are you going to give it? First of all you need to identify the species and discover whether it is by nature vegetarian (eating greenstuffs), granivorous (eating grain and seeds), insectivorous (eating insects), carnivorous (eating meat), piscivorous (eating fish) or effectively omnivorous (eating just about anything it can find, whether animal or vegetable). Appendix 3 gives a full breakdown of birds' natural food preferences: for more detail check a good field guide.

The shape of a bird's beak is a major clue to its feeding preferences. Carnivores that tear flesh have strong, short, hooked beaks, whereas insectivores have thin, delicate ones (like the robin) or stronger ones for hammering into bark to extract grubs, or a wide gape to catch flying insects (swifts etc.). Specialist fish-eaters have long, strong, stabbing beaks, but waders or soil-probers have long, thin ones. Dabbling ducks and grazers have broad, flat beaks. Birds that eat a lot of grain and seeds have fairly stout, hard beaks to crack their food (for example, finches and sparrows). Omnivores and opportunist feeders like gulls, crows and tits have all-purpose beaks best suited to their environment.

The terms "hardbill" and "softbill" are often used by aviculturists to differentiate song-birds not according to the texture of their beaks but to the type of food they eat. A hardbill is a vegetarian who enjoys a wide variety of weed seeds and has a bill tough enough to crack grains and nuts, and the group includes birds like finches and buntings; a softbill is carnivorous, eating things like worms, caterpillars and grubs, and the group includes thrushes, blackbirds, robins, starlings, and so on. Hardbills are easily catered for: they will eat seeds and peanuts. The softbills are a little more difficult but can make do with ox heart, cheese and scrambled or hard-boiled egg until you can acquire some proprietary insectivorous food or get juicy morsels like mealworms.

Ideally you would try and offer the bird the kind of food it would choose for itself in the wild, according to the present season, but it is most unlikely that you will be able to do so, however hard you try and however much time you have to spare. So you will have to compromise. Suitable alternatives to a bird's natural food preferences are also given, species by species, in Appendix 3. Birds of prey, however, have rather special feeding requirements and it is best to hand them over to an expert.

The essence of feeding wildlife (and it should also apply to domesticated or permanently confined creatures of all kind) is to offer a wide variety of foods, so that deficiencies in one kind can be counterbalanced by another. This is particularly the case with most birds, which in the wild eat little helpings of lots of different foods.

FEEDING MAMMALS

Variety and ingenuity are equally important in considering food for mammals, as is the need to identify the species and then ascertain its natural diet, the time at which it would normally eat and the frequency of its meals. Appendix 3 contains a species-by-species guide to natural food preferences of mammals and suitable alternatives.

Many carnivorous and insectivorous mammals will do well enough on tinned dogmeat or perhaps catfood. If a carnivore is given fresh, raw meat it will definitely need supplementary vitamins and minerals in the absence of those it would naturally find in the bones, offal, brains, gut contents and fur or feathers of its prey. If you want to feed whole carcases, either regularly or occasionally, go for the invaluable day-old chicks (if they can still be found) or pinkies, or pick up RTA corpses as long as you are absolutely certain they have not been poisoned or otherwise contaminated and are very fresh. If you have a large freezer, it can be invaluable for stocking up all these sources of food but they must be thoroughly thawed before being fed to your patient.

FEEDING AMPHIBIANS AND REPTILES

Frogs and toads are carnivores: they like all kinds of invertebrates. Up to 25 per cent of a frog's diet is usually slugs and snails, whereas a toad enjoys ants (40 per cent), beetles (15 per cent) and woodlice (15 per cent), and a natterjack toad eats enormous numbers of fly larvae (especially crane flies) which might make up to 30 per cent of its diet. All of them also eat woodlice, beetles, millipedes, centipedes, spiders, flies, moths, butterflies, caddis flies, earwigs, bugs, springtails and even bees, but not wasps or hairy caterpillars.

Earthworms are greatly relished, particularly by the common toad.

Tadpoles are omnivorous and can live on a largely vegetarian diet if necessary. Most of their food is algae and protozoa (tiny water animals) but they also occasionally eat carrion, spawn and each other. In captivity they can be fed boiled lettuce or the type of pellets you can buy in pet shops for rabbits and hamsters.

Snakes are generally carnivorous with quite catholic tastes in the wild. In captivity they will enjoy a freshly dead mouse, day-old chicks and insect larvae, but they are spasmodic eaters and do not need regular feeding. Most snakes only need a meal perhaps three times a week, or even once a week. Adders rarely eat in captivity, though they might be tempted by mice and chicks.

Slow-worms feed in the late afternoon and early evening, and enjoy slugs, snails, insects and worms, while most of the other lizards will eat insects and also like fruit and lettuce.

Tortoises will eat almost any plant in the garden—grass, vegetables, weeds and of course ornamental bedding plants! **Terrapins**, however, are active fish-hunters.

FOODSTUFFS AND HOW TO ADMINSTER THEM

Foods of Animal Origin

Day-old hatchery chicks   These are surplus male chicks available from hatcheries which produce egg-laying pullets. Choose your source with care, in view of salmonella contamination within the industry. The chicks, still full of egg-food after hatching, are a very good source of food for raptors and carnivorous mammals. Use freshly killed, or store in a freezer immediately and thaw thoroughly before feeding. Feed whole for roughage and minerals as well as meat. To tempt a bird of prey not used to dead food, try quartering the chick to expose its innards.

Laboratory rodents   "Pinkies" are naked new-born rodents, or you can use older animals as long as they have not been experimentally fed or injected. Albino mice are also reared commercially for sale to pet shops and aviculturists, or you could breed your own in metal cages in a warm room (say 24 °C): mice are sexually mature at only two months old and, with a gestation period of only nineteen days, a female might produce eight litters a year with perhaps half a dozen in each litter.

Feed like day-old chicks—either freshly killed, or thoroughly thawed after deep-freezing.

Road Traffic Accidents (RTAs) Corpses on the road are useful food provided they are very fresh and not diseased, poisoned or otherwise contaminated.

Raw meat Can be fed in strips or minced but *must* be judiciously supplemented with minerals and vitamins if given to true carnivores as their only food. Add an appropriate powdered supplement in measured amounts sprinkled on the meat, perhaps with coat combings from your dog or cat, for roughage. Moisten meat before offering to raptors, who rarely drink water as they normally find enough moisture in their food. Avoid feeding raw pork and be careful with raw poultry meat.

Ox heart and liver Often better foods (and cheaper) than raw beef and can be used for a wide range of animals. Liver is an excellent appetiser: many creatures will take liver even when refusing other food. However, do not use liver as a staple food—feed it perhaps three times a week as a supplement to raw meat.

Eggs Very useful food for many animals and particularly for birds. Do not give too often to mammals, although most of them adore raw eggs. Can be fed raw, scrambled, or hard-boiled and then chopped or grated.

Milk Beware: milk is not a natural food for adult mammals and certainly not for birds, amphibians and reptiles. It can cause quite severe and dangerous digestive upset and diarrhoea, especially if it is cow's milk. Sheep and goat's milk, especially the latter, are more digestible and (unlike cow's) can be frozen for storage, but in general you should *not* give milk to adults—and that includes hedgehogs.

Cheese Cottage cheese is a useful standby, or a little grated Cheddar to whet an appetite. Be careful with salted cheese (most hard cheeses): most creatures should not be given salted foods.

Tinned petfood Tinned dogmeat or catfood are useful in emergencies and are already fortified with minerals and vitamins, unlike raw meat. But feed with care and watch the effects of any particular brand on the patient's digestive system. The more expensive brands sometimes give very loose droppings. Mustelids usually do better on a cheap cereal-based brand like Chappie, though it makes their droppings a funny colour! Can be offered to most carnivores and many birds, including insectivores, but be wary of long-term use.

Fish and seafood Fish for piscivores should be fed raw and very fresh indeed, or frozen while very fresh and then thoroughly thawed for immediate feeding. Most fish-eating birds prefer whole fish offered head first (slides down the throat easier that way round) but you could also offer strips of larger white fish. Possibilities include, above all, sprats, also whitebait, cod strips, mackerel, herring, smelt, sardine, mullet, anchovy, depending on what is locally available. Choose a size of fish suitable to size of bird. Dead fish lose their thiamin content almost immediately: if you feed dead rather than live fish, consider the need for supplements, especially vitamin E for frozen fish. In emergencies you could use tinned catfood containing fish, tinned fish-purée baby foods, or tinned salmon, pilchards and sardines, but not drowned in oil. Shrimps are good, too.

Insect Foods

Insects are eaten at all stages of their life cycles by many birds and also by reptiles, amphibians and some mammals. Collecting from the wild will be time-consuming and laborious, and may or may not be appreciated by your patients. If you do collect live insects (for example, by using a sweep-net among shrubbery or under a tree branch which is tapped with a stick to shake out insects) beware of plants which have been sprayed with pesticides. Flying insects can be captured in special insect-traps, usually with the aid of an attractive source of light, and some people instal light-bulbs above an outdoor aviary for that purpose. Many grubs and caterpillars are relished by insectivores but many are not, and you might find you have collected the inedible or poisonous rather than the desirable. Beware of hairy caterpillars, for example, and take great care with "gentles" or fly maggots which are probably full of the putrefied food they have been eating. A well-loved delicacy for many insectivores is ants' eggs—look under paving stones on sand, for example. Most insect eggs and grubs are found under stones or leaves, in bark crevices or under rotting bark, or on specific host plants, so get probing and turning things over! Do try and give live insect food to insectivores at least occasionally to vary their diet and give them something to stimulate their interest: you can buy live food from commercial sources (though this is an expensive option) or create your own breeding colony of suitable insects which can be harvested as grubs or as adults. The alternative is to buy proprietary insectivorous foods but choose them carefully; different mixtures suit different species. The best of the avian products are also useful for shrews, hedgehogs, moles and bats, and possibly some amphibians and reptiles. The names and addresses of some of the major manufacturers and suppliers of insectivorous foods are to be found in Appendix 6.

Foods of Vegetable Origin

Peanuts   Peanuts are not actually nuts: they are legumes. They are an excellent source of protein, much enjoyed by a wide range of birds and mammals. However, they should be fed with caution: too many can be fattening, as they contain a high proportion of oil. They should also be purchased with caution: kept in damp conditions they are susceptible to a mould which gives rise to unpleasant and often fatal respiratory diseases. Only buy from a reliable source, preferably one which can guarantee their peanuts are free from aflatoxin fungi. Feed peanut kernels whole or crushed, but never salted.

Wild nuts   Many wild nuts and tree seeds are appreciated by birds and mammals, including acorns, beechmast and hazel nuts in particular. Sweet chestnut is liked by some, but horse chestnut is rarely popular, though it can be ground into a flour. Acorns can be boiled and mashed for poultry, but can be poisonous to livestock if eaten in any quantity, though livestock often develop a perverse craving for them. Beechmast is a good source of protein. Almonds (not salted, and certainly not sugar-coated) are also useful, as are pine kernels.

Seeds   There is a huge range of seeds suitable for birds, and there is ample scope for collecting wild seed or "cultivating" your own. Important bird seeds (often available from pet shops) include hemp, millet, canary seed, niger and of course sunflower seeds, which are adored by a wide variety of birds and rodents.

If you are collecting seeds from the wild, make absolutely certain the plants have not been sprayed with insecticides or weed-killer: it is safer to let the plants grow in your own garden and you should always make space for that essential wild plant, chickweed, which gives the best of greenfoods as well as its seeds. You might also grow shepherd's purse, plantains, a little groundsel (but it might give loose droppings), various meadow grasses and knotgrasses, poppies, rape, flax, teazel (a favourite of some finches, and a handsome, tall plant in the garden or field) and sowthistle. Several of the weeds also supply valuable greenfood.

Note that poppy, rape, niger, flax, hemp, sesame and sunflower seeds have a high fat content. Top of the protein tables are peanuts, flax, hemp, caraway, poppy, sesame, niger and rape. Sunflower seeds and canary seed have a high fibre content.

Also useful is Trill, the seed mixture that, apart from its quality and good supply of additives, is available at your local supermarket.

Grains   The standard grains available from feed merchants and pet shops are wheat and maize. You could also use buckwheat, soybean and boiled unsalted brown rice.

Grain and grassmeal often form the basis of various poultry and pheasant pellets, which are usually sold by feed merchants according to the bird's stage of development (rearing, layers, breeders etc.). Turkey grower pellets seem to be suitable for birds like peacocks and guineafowl. But you should be aware that pellets contain all sorts of additives, some of which might be inappropriate: check the ingredients carefully.

Grain is also the basis of bread, cereals, dog biscuits and puppy meal, all of which have their place in feedstuffs. Avoid feeding fresh bread to any creature: use stale or dried bread and give free access to drinking water. Also avoid white bread in favour of wholemeal. True carnivores, like raptors and the smaller mustelids, are unable to digest carbohydrate: if they are fed with grain-based food, therefore, it must be thoroughly cooked.

Berries and fruit   Fruit is an essential part of the diet for some birds and an enjoyment for many other birds and mammals. Useful fresh fruits include apple, cherry, grape, banana, plum, melon and avocado. Dried fruits are good standby rations but need to be soaked in water overnight before being fed. The range of berries is considerable, embracing cultivated fruit-garden berries, ornamental shrub berries and wild berries, and it should be possible to find suitable ripe berries at most times of year—or you could try freezing, drying or bottling some by way of experiment.

Green food and vegetables   For wild birds, some of the weeds provide an important source of green food, especially chickweed, dandelion, shepherd's purse, sowthistle, watercress and groundsel (choose the tender tips).

Garden greens include spinach and lettuce, but if you buy these in, be very suspicious, especially with lettuce: many growers spray them with pesticides and fungicides, and many a bird has died from eating lettuce for that reason. Crops like cabbage, swiss chard, alfalfa and lucerne all have their place in feeding, and above all of them comes comfrey, a rampant perennial plant rich in protein, carbohydrates and minerals, and an excellent food not only for birds but also for grazing animals. It is the only plant known to extract vitamin B12 from the soil and it is also a good source of calcium.

The most useful greenfood of all must be grass. Young grass is a highly nutritious and well balanced food for creatures which have the ability to digest it—it is ideal for grazing animals, rabbits and hares, and swans and geese. Where possible the animal should be allowed to graze growing grass, or given freshly cut clippings, and waterfowl pens benefit from being planted with a mixed sward of wheat, oats, barley and rye so that the birds can graze the growing shoots. An alternative where grazing is not available is to grow hydroponic "grass", which is very young growths of cereal plants and, like young grass, is highly nutritious and full of proteins, vitamins and minerals. Basically, you sow oats or barley grains on plastic trays and spray them every six to eight hours with water containing plant nutrients. Keep the surroundings at a constant 17 °C to 19 °C and under continuous fluorescent lighting. The system is similar in principle to kitchen bean-sprouts, another good source of nutrition.

Many fresh garden vegetables have a role to play—for example, carrots, sweetcorn, tomatoes, runner beans, peas and cucumber. Dried lentils appeal to some birds if they are soaked overnight and lightly boiled to make them soft.

Water plants   Make the most of pondweed for swans and duckweed for ducks, complete with their colonies of molluscs and insect life.

Supplements

Vitamins and minerals   Be cautious about adding vitamin and mineral supplements to an animal's ration. It should be possible to provide enough variety in the diet to ensure a good balance of vitamins and minerals, and this is preferable to supplements. Both deficiencies and excesses can have a considerable effect on an animal's health and you need to be aware that fat-soluble vitamins (A, D, E and K) given in excess are not easily removed from the animal's system and can therefore be toxic.

Two of the most important minerals are calcium and phosphorus, which are complementary, and the balance between them plays a major role. Deficiencies in these elements can be a considerable problem for captive wildlife and domestic animals. Good sources of calcium include sardines, some insects, snail-shells, egg-shells, bones, grasses, dry alfalfa, fungi, soybean and sunflower seeds; good phosphorus sources include sardines, liver, barley, wheat, oats, acorns, soybean and sunflower seeds. The most useful calcium supplements are bonemeal (but do not buy it from a garden shop), limestone and shell (oyster, egg or snail). However, to make use of these sources the animal also needs adequate vitamin D, the "sunshine" vitamin. Sunshine is free: take full advantage of it.

Raw meat is very deficient in calcium, which is one good reason for feeding whole carcases to carnivores at least three times a week. Meat is also deficient in some other minerals—for example, iodine, a deficiency of which can lead to the development of goitres. Liver, on the other hand, is a good source of iodine and many other minerals and vitamins, including vitamin E, which is lacking in red meat.

Another important mineral is salt, or sodium chloride. Birds have a low sodium requirement and should not be given salted foods as it is difficult for them to excrete excess salt. Seabirds are exceptions: their systems are adjusted to a saline environment and they sometimes need the addition of a little salt in their diet in captivity if they do not have access to salt water. The same applies to marine mammals. Terrestrial mammals tend to find enough salt naturally in their food, especially carnivores. Rabbits have perfected the art of recycling their own droppings to extract sodium. Grazing animals on sodium-deficient pasture need a mineral lick, obtainable from livestock suppliers, and a sure sign of such a deficiency is when an animal will lick *anything* for salt, including treated wooden structures, bonfire ash and even urine-soaked soil.

Supplements *do* have a role to play but should not be used at random. They are particularly important at certain stages in an animal's life: for example, during early growth and during breeding and, in the case of birds, during feather regrowth after the moult. The aim should always be to give a creature a choice from a wide range of foods and trust it to select what it really needs, making sure at the same time that it does not simply choose to stuff itself with its favourite tit-bit, especially if that tit-bit is something it would have access to in its wild state.

Commercial "complete" foods   Complan is a highly nutritious "complete" food designed for human invalids and infants but it has also saved the life of many an animal casualty. It is good for an anorexic animal or one needing a light diet, or for post-operative cases. Cats prefer it more diluted, and different animals have different preferences which you will only discover by trial and error. Complan is based on powdered skimmed milk and its manufacturers also make Farex, which is not milk-based and may be more suitable in some cases.

Mazuri Zoo Foods cater for a wide range of species and they offer special diets for waterfowl, pheasants, bovines, ungulates, sheep, equines, rodents, pigs, guinea-pigs, lagomorphs, primates, carnivores, amphibians—you name it! Their products are not available in small quantities but their Special Diets Service is always willing to give advice on feeding different species, and you might be able to liaise with a zoo to obtain supplies.

John Cooper's insectivore mix   John Cooper, a leading veterinary surgeon with considerable knowledge, especially with wildlife, suggests the following emergency home mix for small insectivores in his classic book, *First Aid and Care of Wild Birds*:

Use any cereal product as a base. Add some or all of the following: soya flour or ground soybeans, honey, grated Cheddar cheese, lightly steamed liver, grated carrot, celery, currants, raw cabbage, figs, dates, apple, nuts or peanut butter, dried milk and powdered baby or invalid food (Farex); you could also add leftover roast beef or sausages, fresh fish heads, prawns or sardines, minced up and mixed into the basic ingredients. Make the whole lot into a light, crumbly mixture and add a multi-vitamin supplement like Abidec (liquid in drinking water) or Vionate (powder in food). Put a couple of live mealworms on top of the food to catch the bird's attention.

CHAPTER EIGHT

ORPHANS

There is something irresistible about a young, helpless creature who seems to have no friend in the world but you and who seems to look to you as its saviour. It is that very helplessness which encourages the parents of the new-born to care for it—to feed it, keep it warm, and protect it from predators and the elements, often at considerable personal expense.

This is a hard act for a human foster parent to follow. If you are tempted to try, be warned that you have every chance of failing. If you do experience the magical joy of success, what happens then to the orphan that has outgrown you but perhaps half believes it is human?

Sometimes parents reject an offspring for good reason, perhaps mental weakness or a fatal physical problem, so that your help might be to no avail—but you can still try. You will probably fail, but you can learn from failure so that you can do better next time and can share your experience with others as well. However, for the sake of the animals, you should pass the young of certain species—especially otters, seals and birds of prey—to specialists.

In the opening chapters, warnings were given about assuming a young wild creature found alone has been abandoned and the warnings must be repeated in this chapter. In the great majority of cases, that little thing is not an orphan at all and your interference is both unwelcome and potentially disastrous.

ORPHAN BIRDS

If you find a young, feathered bird sitting on your lawn or hopping about looking faintly lost and lonely, it is very likely that its parents are either elsewhere gathering food for it or are watching from cover, waiting for you to go away. So, unless the fledgling is in danger from cats and cars or is obviously injured or sick, go away. And keep away—or at least out of sight—for a couple of hours.

Do not try and put a feathered bird back in its nest. Several species, especially owls, leave the nest before they can fly and are fed by their parents until they can look after themselves. If you are worried about predators, put the bird in shrubbery out of reach but in a place where the parents can easily find and feed it (its persistent calling will draw them). You could also put it in an open box or cage, as long as the parents can feed it easily, and then put the container out of cat reach in a bush so that it is protected from heavy rain and direct sunlight—preferably as near the nest as possible, if you know where that is, but without disturbing the rest of the brood if they are still in the nest, or you may precipitate a sudden, explosive and possibly premature departure. If it is late in the day, the bird could be brought indoors overnight to keep it warm but it must be put out again at dawn so that the parent can feed it.

In some situations, however, you will be justified in taking more positive action. If the little bird is not feathered, it is a nestling rather than a fledgling and does need to be replaced in its nest—*its* nest—though it might have been ejected for good reason and will soon be pushed out again. In that case its only hope of survival is under your care.

Likewise, if it is a fledgling and the parents do not return to feed it after a couple of hours, if it is suffering in some way, or if you have found it at dusk with a crop which does not feel full, it needs help. Think very hard about whether you can or should try to rear it yourself. You will need a great deal of time, patience and luck to succeed, and with feeding on an hourly or two-hourly basis from dawn to dusk in the early days it is essential that someone reliable is at home all the time—for several weeks if necessary, seven days a week. Nestlings will need more concentrated attention than fledglings and will have to remain in your care longer, but they might be easier to deal with because fledglings are much more aware of what is happening to them and will be in shock from such close contact with humans. They will be unable to feed themselves' but will be under stress at being fed by you.

There is much more to orphan rearing than offering the right accommodation, keeping it warm, finding the right food, persuading the bird to eat it, keeping it clean and keeping it healthy. Right from the first moment you have to think of its whole future and prepare it so that it will be able to fend for itself in its natural environment and live (and breed) among its own kind. It is perhaps the rehabilitation aspect which is the most difficult to manage. You might decide to hand the orphan to those who are experienced but they will already be overwhelmed with similar cases. Your thoughts might turn to a local aviculturist, but wild birds should really be kept away from cage and aviary birds for fear of introducing parasites and disease.

So think hard before you make your decision and do not act on impulse. Do not start unless you are prepared to go all the way to independence. If it is a bird of prey, think even harder. It will be fairly easy to rear but has special needs and could be quite difficult to rehabilitate, and what is more its parents, if they are still around, will probably attack you quite viciously if you try and pick up their offspring.

FOSTERING

It might be possible for a nestling to be fostered by another bird. If so, the bird will make a much better parent than you could ever be and the little one will never be confused about its own identity as a bird. Some birds, especially birds of prey and chicks, ducklings and goslings, quickly become imprinted when they are very young and identify with their "parent". Imprinting can last a lifetime, so that an orphan gosling reared by hand or fostered on a mother hen might never be able to relate to another goose or mate successfully with its own species. In the case of raptors which you hope to rehabilitate in due course, or disabled ones retained for captive breeding, you should resist the temptation to stroke them and should not even talk to them: you should not exist for them and should try to devise ways of feeding them so that they never associate you with food. It will be difficult: you will long for them to recognise you and respond to you but that would not be in their long-term interests.

The mainstay of the barnyard, the broody hen, has for centuries played the role of foster mother to all sort of chicks, ducklings, goslings and cygnets. She will make an excellent job of rearing them though she might find their unchickenlike behaviour worrying and she will cluck about them fussily in typical hen fashion. But she knows how to keep them warm, she knows how to encourage them to feed themselves and she knows how to teach them about the dangerous world around them. If you have a good broody at the right moment, especially a Silkie, make full use of her to rear ducks, geese, swans, pheasants, peafowl, turkeys and guineafowl. However, she will be no use at all for birds of prey, nor is she appropriate for the smaller nest-reared species which are the birds most likely to come into your care. Although she will scratch about to find food, she expects her young to feed themselves and will not understand what all that gaping is for.

The ubiquity of blue and great tits in the garden means that many parent birds are caught by cats or sparrow hawks, so that many orphan fledglings will be tits. John Goodman, warden of the RSPCA Mallydams wildlife centre on the Sussex coast near Hastings, is in the happy position of having a woodland bird sanctuary as well as a rescue centre and field centre, so that if he finds an orphaned nestling blue tit he knows exactly where a dozen other blue tits are nesting and he can sneak the orphan into a nestbox with another brood of the same age and size. A hand-reared nestling just getting to the active stage is an ideal candidate for this kind of placement. The foster parents cannot count and will usually accept the newcomer without noticing. Then the orphan will be raised on the right sort of food and among its own kind, leaving the box with the rest of the brood when the time is right and remaining part of a family group so that it learns to respond to dangers and social situations and is accustomed to its natural habitat.

There are dangers in this attractive idea. For a start, it is illegal to disturb any wild bird's nest. In more practical terms, a nest should not be overloaded with young: the number must relate to the amount of food available in the parent birds' environment. Also, beware of causing the emergence of the resident brood: do not put an orphan into a nest when the brood is only a few days away from leaving home or you could precipitate a premature evacuation.

Some rescue centres have disabled birds of prey as permanent residents because they are unable to fend for themselves in the wild, and these birds are used as foster parents for appropriate species, overcoming the problem of human imprinting. However, this type of fostering needs careful and experienced supervision by people who understand the ways of birds of prey and who have a licence to keep them.

HAND-REARING

When fostering is not a possibility, you will have to hand-rear your bird. First of all, identify the species. Broadly, is it a chick, that is, a *nidifugous* or precocial species, and if so is it of the kind which is able to feed itself as soon as it leaves the nest (for example, ducklings, goslings, gamebird chicks) or one that leaves the nest within hours of hatching but has to be fed by its parents (moorhen, coot, heron etc.)? Or is it a *nidicolous* species which remains on the nest and is fed there until it fledges, when it will still be fed for a while by its parents until it learns to find its own food? Or is it a bird of prey which is likely to depend on its parents for food for quite a long time? Chicks are downy when they hatch—they have to be ready to go straight out into the world—but one chick looks very like another, though it is easy enough to tell wildfowl (ducks, geese, swans) from game chicks, or from rail chicks which are basically black rather than yellow and brown, and have huge unwebbed feet. Nidicolous or altricial birds are unfeathered for quite a while until they are fledglings, and it can be very difficult to identify the actual species but you should make every effort to do so in order to feed it appropriately in due course.

ACCOMMODATION

Nestlings

Because of their lack of feathers, nestlings need plenty of warmth. During their first ten days of life their accommodation needs to be kept at a steady temperature of 27-32 °C, or even warmer if their eyes are not yet open or if they are an exotic species. Heat loss will be an urgent and immediate problem when you find a nestling: it can lose heat very fast. A warm box in a dark place can work wonders as a first step while you work out something more permanent.

Ideally you should use an abandoned nest (making sure it is free of parasites) or make an artifical nest-pan just a little larger than the bird or brood. For example, use a strawberry punnet or something similar lined with soft, warm materials like old woollen clothing, flannelette nappies or clean socks, and cover with several layers of soft tissue which can be changed frequently to keep the nest clean.

Put the nest into a draught-free container of some kind. You could use a clean, dry aquarium with its own heating system and light, a hospital cage or avicultural drying cage or even a shoe box. Have a piece of flannel to cover the nestling: that will keep it warmer and will also remove the triggers that set off its feed-demanding instincts. Uncover it at feeding time, then cover it again after feeding so that it can sleep.

Unless the container has its own heating system, you need to devise a direct source of heat. A hot-water bottle under the box, insulated with half a dozen layers of newspaper to retain the heat, will be very comforting but will need replacing every few hours. You could rig up a red 40-watt electric light-bulb in an emergency; the bulb needs to be red so that it does not keep the bird awake all night, and if the bird is a hole-nesting species it should in any case be kept in subdued light all the time. You can make your own brooder from a fairly large, stiff cardboard box: there will be plenty of them at the supermarket for free. Cut away half of the lid and tape the other half firmly in place as a partial roof, then cut a hole in the roof to admit the heat from a light-bulb connected to a dimmer switch (which is cheaper than a thermostat) and put the nest under the bulb with a thermometer next to it so that you can keep a check on the temperature of the nest. Use a blanket or towel to cover the open half of the roof to increase the warmth when necessary. If the bird feels too warm under the bulb, it has the option of moving to the cooler, open-topped half of the box. (An overheated bird lies with its legs and wings stretched out; too cold a bird huddles up or wanders about cheeping to itself.)

When the bird becomes more adventurous, turn the box into a cage by cutting a window in the side and covering it with fine-mesh Twilweld, so that the bird has a view of the outside world. Stimulate its interest further by putting a "play" platform in the box, scattered with a few leafless hazel or apple twigs. It will begin to pick up the twigs experimentally and this can be the first step towards self-feeding: scatter some powdered cuttlefish or very fine grit on the platform with some freshly crushed millet seed if it is a seed-eating species, and place a shallow water dish on the platform too. When the bird seems to want to get out of its box, it is ready to be transferred to a cage with a low perch in it and is almost ready to be given enough space to practise flying.

Fledglings

Fledglings need less heat as their feathers begin to develop. When well-feathered, they need artificial heat only in cold weather, though they should be covered at night and should be kept out of draughts at all times. Newly arrived fledglings can be popped into a cardboard box with its base lined with thick layers of newspaper, which should be changed at least daily.

Chicks

The down on chicks is not adequate protection and in the early stages they need continuous warmth, gradually reducing in temperature and duration as they develop. If they have just hatched, they are at considerable risk of heat loss until they have dried off from the egg.

An infra-red poultry or gamebird brooder is ideal for a group of chicks (see Fig. 39 on p. 128). Make a circular pen out of strong cardboard or panels of hardboard to protect them from draughts, and give them a dummy "mother" for comfort—something they can hide under, perhaps with cloth strips masquerading as motherly feathers, or a dry mophead. Rail chicks *must* have a place where they can hide from you—they are very nervous of humans. Gradually reduce the artificial heat until the birds are feathered and ready to go out of doors in something like a portable chicken ark. Ducklings need to go outside as soon as possible because they will develop much better, but they do need access to shelter from heavy rain and hot sun even when they have been hardened off. Do not use newspaper floor covering for ducks at any stage—they cannot keep their balance and will develop deformed limbs—but use something like sawdust, cloths or paper towels. If they are to be released into the wild, try and leave the birds alone as much as possible so that they do not become "humanised".

Birds of Prey

Raptors do not need artificial heat and can usually be kept quite simply in a draught-free cardboard or wooden box. Do not use newspaper on the floor: it is too slippery for them and they will soon develop splayed legs. Try and give them some thick twigs to perch on if they wish. Their instinct will be to defecate over the edge of the nest to keep it clean, if they can. Do not allow them to bathe until their down has been replaced by proper feathering.

WATER

Nestlings should be able to get all the moisture they need from their food but fledglings should have a shallow bowl of fresh drinking water within reach: make sure they cannot tip it over or drown in it. Chicks need drinking water right from the start; for the first few days this can be a shallow dish with some pebbles in it to make sure they cannot drown and some coloured marbles to draw their attention to the water. Then gradually train them to use poultry drinkers (or an inverted jam jar on a saucer) so that they cannot foul the water or climb into it. Do not let waterfowl chicks take a bath until their breasts are properly feathered. However, they will need to be able to get their heads in water now and then to keep their eyes healthy and their bills and nostrils clean, and they will do their utmost to bathe from a very early age.

FEEDING

Now for the difficult part. This is where you need lots of time, patience, ingenuity and Tender Loving Care. Young birds need feeding right through the day, from dawn to dusk—hourly to start with—though you will probably find it better to adjust the bird to your own routines to some extent by feeding in the evening and giving a last feed at about 11 p.m. so that you do not have to rise with the dawn.

There are no immutable rules about how to feed but the following suggestions are based on the experience of many people over many years. The first few feeds will be the most difficult but after that both you and the orphan will be more in tune with each other and fall into a mutually acceptable routine. Be prepared, therefore, to take a lot of time and care with the first feeds and to do all you can to reduce trauma. Be very gentle, keep all your movements slow and predictable, and talk as much friendly nonsense to the bird as you like. Keep all the feeding equipment scrupulously clean, including your own hands, and also clean up the bird after feeding, using damp cottonwool and then drying it thoroughly.

Nestlings

Nestlings need to be fed once an hour during daylight. If they are less than about two weeks old, most will automatically "gape", opening their beaks wide in expectation of food. Older nestlings might need encouragement for the first two or three feeds. Once a young bird does gape, it will feed to capacity and then stop gaping.

For the first feed, sit on the floor so that if the bird escapes it will not have far to fall. Hold the bird gently in one hand and use a feeding implement in the other to ease the beak open carefully by introducing the tip of the implement at the side of the beak near the hinge. Then push a little food into its mouth but not *too* little: there should be enough to make the bird swallow. People have personal preferences in the choice of implement: try a tiny spoon, or the flat end of a small wooden spatula, the tip of an artist's brush, a piece of small-diameter plastic tubing, a plastic 3 cc syringe which you can get from your vet, or a long, narrow pair of blunt-ended forceps. Obviously the consistency of the feedstuff dictates to some extent what implement you use.

Rather than force-feeding, try a few tricks by thinking bird. For example, a gull reacts to a red spot on the parental bill above its head, which stimulates it to peck at the spot so that the parent then regurgitates half-digested fish in front of it. Baby gulls can be easily fooled by even the crudest imitation bill, as long as that red spot is there so that the urge to feed is triggered. Also think of how the parent would approach the nest. Many fly from *under* the nestling's eye-level and suddenly appear over the edge of the nest; others appear at an entrance hole and the blocking off of light triggers the nestling's gape reaction to imminent feeding. Some birds give a special call as they approach the nest and if you can imitate the right sound it might help to stimulate a reluctant gaper—but make sure you are giving it the right message! Most nestlings will be alarmed if your hand approaches them from above like a predator. If you can succeed in encouraging the bird to gape in its nest so that it is not actually handled, then so much the better.

Nestlings can eat the equivalent of their own weight in food every day and the smaller the species the more frequently it needs feeding. Be responsive to the bird's demands, but also beware of letting it get crop-bound. If the crop is still full at the next feed, there is a digestive problem which needs to be sorted out. Sometimes a bird needs to be winded like a human baby if you have managed to let it swallow air, and you can gently work the air bubble up out of its crop from the base upwards by massaging it so that you can feel the bubble's progress.

Little and often is the best for most nestlings and they will not overeat. Stop feeding when they stop gaping or when they seem to hold the last offering of food in their mouths rather than swallowing it down. The last feed of the evening is an important one: the bird needs a full crop to see it through the night.

The immediate reaction of most young birds to the stimulus of food is to eject a dropping, which should be removed at once in order to keep the nest clean. Always keep the bird clean of its own food as well.

Fledglings

Fledglings can be more difficult to persuade to feed than nestlings. Their responses are not so automatic and they are more individual in their reactions. An active fledgling should soon learn to feed itself and at that stage it needs constant access to fresh food in a dish. Be ingenious in encouraging early independent feeding as part of the rehabilitation programme. Birds are adept at learning by example from similar species, and a tame canary in a separate cage in full view of a finch fledgling will soon encourage it to imitate appropriate eating habits.

The explosive feather growth at this stage needs enormous resources of energy in the fledgling and it is vital that the food is highly nutritious and available in adequate quantities. Poor feeding can give the bird severe plumage defects later, with stress fractures across the feather, and in a flight feather that could be dangerous. Fledglings need a very high proportion of protein in their diet, and in the wild the parents positively cram their young with the richest sources of animal protein they can find.

It is essential to keep the developing feathers uncontaminated by droppings. At the fledgling stage the viscid faecal sacs ejected during feeding should be caught before they burst (use a pair of tweezers) and this can be quite a juggling act if there is more than one bird to feed in a nest. Once they become active, the sac becomes a normal dropping and some foods, especially tinned dogmeat, make the droppings messily liquid. Another potential though fairly rare problem at this stage is neck ballooning during feeding in some species and sometimes the balloon needs to be pricked carefully with a sterile needle. Then there is the rubbery beak which some fledglings, especially blackbirds, seem to develop: the beak becomes so soft that the bird cannot take down its food. This seems to be connected with the huge demands made by feather production and fast body growth at this time.

Before it can be released, a fledgling needs to be gradually weaned off hand-feeding completely so that it learns to feed itself. With most birds, begin to introduce live food like mealworms in a container on top of the usual food; this should stimulate their interest and encourage them to help themselves. Phase out the hand-feeding gradually because you do not want to reduce the bird's overall intake of nutrition.

Chicks

Chicks are easier to deal with in a brood than as individuals and an orphan will be much happier with others of its own age and size, even if they are of different species. Gamekeepers often use a more "experienced" chick—perhaps a duckling a couple of days older than a batch of pheasant chicks—to set an example to the newcomers and teach them about food and drink. A lone chick will be suffering from shock: its development is so advanced immediately after hatching that it is much more aware of its environment than, say, a passerine nestling. Whereas a blue tit nestling is touchingly trusting, it will probably be quite difficult to gain a lone chick's confidence: it will panic and start rushing around in agitation when you try and feed it. The aim is to encourage it to self-feed from the start and perhaps the best method with a reluctant feeder is to put down a very shallow dish of food, dip an artist's brush in it and transfer a blob of the food on to the bird's plumage. It will then start preening itself and discover *food!* With luck it will soon be helping itself from the dish. It will be more attracted if you put something eye-catching on top of the food like a wriggling maggot or mealworm, or make the food seem to be alive by letting a couple of drops of water fall on it. Another trick is to lay a trail of food scattered on the ground and leading towards the dish, or scatter some food and then imitate a hen scratching around so that the chick comes to investigate your "tit-bitting".

The more dependent species like rails and grebes will have to be fed like nestlings and you need to consider natural parental behaviour. For example, a coot dangles strands of pondweed in front of its chick in rather a cautious way and the chick takes it from the parent's beak. The rails feed their young continually, often with the help of an earlier brood: it is a ceaseless task and you, too, need to offer dangling food constantly.

Birds of Prey

Raptors have different reactions. Hold the food in blunted forceps and move it up and down in front of the chick to stimulate it to open up so that you can drop the morsel into its mouth. You might have to touch the little bristles at the sides of its beak to stimulate it or, if that fails, gently force food into its mouth for the first few feeds. Soon it will be calling when it is hungry and can be fed to capacity. By the time it is perhaps a month old it will probably be ready to accept food from the floor or placed in its talons, and you should aim to reach this stage as soon as possible. As soon as it is self-feeding, do not let a raptor associate you with food; indeed keep well out of its way. As with other birds, the young raptor can be encouraged to learn self-feeding if an older bird is in sight to show it how.

Be aware that a young raptor eats *much* more than an adult. Offer food four or five times a day, any time—regularity does not matter to a raptor. In the wild the young will have quite long periods without feeding while the parents are hunting for the next meal. They do not need night-feeding, even if they are owls. When they have had enough, they will hold a piece of meat in the beak for quite a while and then drop it.

FOOD

Natural foods are ideal if you know what the natural parent would feed its young at different stages of development and different seasons. Some are very specialist. For example, great tits need endless quantities of those little green tortrix caterpillars that rain from oak trees in May, and they need spiders when they are five to eight days old. Insects are an excellent source of protein for growing birds and easy to digest as well. However, you are unlikely to have the parents' knowledge, nor are you likely to be able to collect wild food fast enough to keep up with an orphan's demands. A dedicated aviculturist spent three hours hunting in his garden for spiders for a young bird and only found half a dozen, though the bird could happily have eaten fifty.

It will probably be more convenient and efficient to devise your own orphan food, which needs to be easy to digest, of the highest quality ingredients, and containing adequate protein but not too much fibre. Eggs and ox heart are excellent emergency rations: the eggs can be scrambled, or hardboiled and then sieved, grated or mashed and mixed with four times as much digestive biscuit by weight, moistened to make a crumbly mixture with an added vitamin supplement, and you can also give some thin slivers of ox heart, chopped earthworms, the juicy insides of mealworms, some greenfly (as long as they have not had access to pesticides), chopped green caterpillars if you can find the right species, or ants' eggs. Other more easily obtained possibilities, according to the species of bird, are cage-bird rearing foods from avicultural suppliers and pet shops, moistened commercial insectivorous mixes, or even tinned baby foods containing animal protein.

Here are some ideas for different types of young bird:

Passerines in general   A good eggfood mix as used for rearing canaries, plus ground-up peanuts and sunflower seed. Add chopped earthworms for thrush family. At the age of four to ten days the mixture needs to be very liquid—about the consistency of thin cream with a solids content of 30 per cent. The consistency gradually thickens thereafter. Try standby foods like oat bran and oat germ from health food shops, or baby foods like beef-and-bone broth (good for growing bones but beware of digestive upset). Give the food tepid but not hot, and *keep* it tepid during the feed by using a hot-water bath for the food container. Increase the animal protein content for fledglings: even seed-eaters feed on caterpillars and larvae.

Finch family   Try any canary rearing food (canaries are members of the finch family) or even foster them on to a good canary after they are five days old as long as they have been fed by their own parents during that time. Or give baby cereal mixed in hot water with a pinch of ground millet from a health food shop, liquidised in a blender and sprinkled with sieved or grated hard-boiled egg. Add a sprinkling of ground cuttlefish bone and tiny shreds of greens once a day.

Psittacines   Baby cereal in hot water with egg yolk, powdered milk, honey, oatmeal, apple sauce and mashed banana, with ground cuttlefish bone. You could add sunflower meal or strained tinned babyfood vegetables. Or beef-and-bone babyfood broth with mixed fruit and nectar (two heaped teaspoons of glucose, one of malt, two of fruit Milupa, mixed with water to make up half a pint) fed moist and tepid. Give weekly vitamin supplement. Stop feeding when the crop feels full. For amazon or cockatoo, add a little bone flour and ground sunflower seed. Wean on to nectar with ground sunflower, gradually coarsening the texture until the bird will accept the seeds whole. Beware of giving fruit eaters too much fruit or greens.

Corvids   Boiled rice, mashed potato, scrambled egg, fruit, wholemeal bread, raw meat, cottage cheese, soaked dog biscuit, insects, chopped mice, ground-up crickets. Dip the food in water and put it well down the throat as the mother would: push the food down with your finger (don't worry, the closing of the beak will not take your finger off). These birds eat a *lot* and are rarely fussy about their food.

Swallow family   Cottage cheese and fresh egg yolk or scrambled egg plus fine dietary grit and vitamin supplement, fed hourly with a teaspoon. Also mealworms or fresh minced meat.

Birds of Prey   Meat, meat, meat! Strips of raw beef or chicken must be supplemented with vitamins, bonemeal and roughage. Small pieces of mouse or pieces of day-old hatchery chicks until they are big enough to accept pinkies, mice and chicks whole. Give the chicks chopped and dampened at first.

Seabirds   Fish. Feed quite a wet mix at first but with good lumps of fish in it for preference: try a moist mash of raw fish and brown bread with a little cod liver oil; graduate to sprats later. Put water next to the food.

Herons   Small eels, small fish, the occasional day-old chick or rodent (chopped up at first).

Ducklings   Grated hard-boiled egg, finely chopped grasses, chick crumbs or mash, insectivorous mix like Sluis Universal, moist chopped sprats and other fish. No pellets for first two weeks. Constant access to drinking/dunking water.

Goslings and Cygnets   Much more vegetarian than ducklings and can take pellets much younger. Give goslings hydroponic grasses, comfrey, kale and other greens, all well shredded, plus soaked biscuit, eggfood and gamebird pellets. Cygnets similar with a whole crumbled hard-boiled egg, including its crushed shell.

Chicks   Pheasant chicks (including peachicks) can have gamebird starter crumbs, shredded lettuce, chickweed, chopped grass, plus egg custard for the first two weeks or crumbled hard-boiled egg later. After two weeks old give two to four mealworms (starved and scalded) or crickets per bird, a little bread and milk, Sluis, vitamin supplements, access to grit/oystershell. Feed guinea keets for first two weeks with crumbled hard-boiled egg with baked corn, fine oatmeal, breadcrumbs, cottage cheese and fine grit; two to six weeks old, gamebird or poultry starter crumbs, shredded lettuce, two to four mealworms or crickets, hard-boiled egg, oyster-shell (chick size); six to twelve weeks old, gamebird pellets, millet seed, chopped alfalfa or hydroponic grasses, oats, hard-boiled egg, insects of all kinds, oyster-shell. Keets are great bug hunters and need more insect food than the pheasant family. Turkey poults can have gamebird or turkey starter crumbs, trout crumbs, hard-boiled egg (yolk only), finely chopped greens like lettuce, dandelion, chickweed or goosegrass (cleavers), insects like mealworms, crickets and beetles, vitamin supplements. Quail chicks feed three times a day (others in this group only need two feeds). Turkey starter meal, hard-boiled egg, a couple of mealworms.

No grit or greens before a week old. Rail and grebe chicks like dangly food—worms, grubs, meat strips, pondweed.

ORPHAN MAMMALS

Mammals, by definition, rear their young on milk and the young are therefore entirely dependent on their mothers until they reach the weaning stage. From then on carnivores will be fed for a considerable time by their parents (and often by other relations) until they have learned to hunt and kill their own food. Thus the rearing of orphan mammals, especially the carnivores, is a long-term job which is likely to be time-consuming and increasingly expensive as the growing animal's appetite increases with its size. With wildlife species, before you decide to try and raise an orphan read the chapters on Rehabilitation and on Law: they might affect your decision. Even before that, remember the warnings about *apparently* abandoned wildlife in earlier chapters. When is an orphan not an orphan? To remind you: deer and hares habitually leave their young "lying up" out in the open, though usually well camouflaged in grass or undergrowth, for many hours at a time, returning to suckle perhaps once or twice a day and spending the rest of the time far afield. Similarly, seals leave their pups on the beach for long periods while they themselves hunt for food at sea. Carnivores necessarily spend a lot of time hunting, usually leaving their young hidden in a more or less permanent den for hours on end, but sometimes the den becomes unsafe and the young are transported to new quarters, one by one and often in stages, and individuals might become stranded for a while during this laborious removal. But they have not been abandoned.

The RSPCA has published an excellent little booklet called *Orphaned Foxes*, whose stated main aim is to "discourage most people from keeping fox cubs, orphaned or otherwise". While comprehensive details of fox-cub management are given, the very strong message of the booklet is, quite simply, *don't*. Do not try to rear a fox as a pet or captive caged animal; do not even start to rear a cub unless you have access to a suitable area for rehabilitation and to a suitable outbuilding and pen, and the ability and desire to make a long-term commitment of several months to prepare the fox for release into the wild. Above all, do not automatically assume that the fox cub you find has been abandoned or is an orphan.

The situations in which you might stumble across a fox cub but should leave it well alone are several. One of them is the change of quarters mentioned above: a cub might be left in the old earth until the following night and on no account should you touch it or the vixen will probably desert it after all. If it seems to be in danger from the cold, give it some bedding in the earth if it is very young; if it is in danger from people and dogs, handle it as little as possible and put it in a box with straw bedding, then slip it back into its earth around dusk so that the vixen can find it. Only if it is still there the following morning should you even consider taking it home and trying to rear it. Remember that, quite apart from the house-moving (which is a common activity during spring), the vixen will not stay in the earth with her cubs during the day except for the first few days of their lives, so that a litter of cubs alone in an earth is unlikely to have been abandoned.

During the summer (perhaps June) the vixen moves her cubs to above-ground lying-up sites like bramble patches, undisturbed wood piles, among grain crops, in barns and outbuildings, or even in urban gardens. In the latter situation, people often assume the cubs are orphans—the little ones might be seen playing in the open with no sign of the mother, who usually comes out only at night. If they really are orphans, they will look rather lost, aimless and plaintive rather than playful or contentedly sleepy, and there will be no sign of food debris anywhere. Sometimes a young cub goes out exploring, like any curious and active young mammal, and might become trapped in a building or fall into a pit or simply get lost and hide somewhere until nightfall. In such a case, it will not be far from home and if it is merely taking shelter you should leave it alone: it will re-establish contact with its family after dusk. If it is in some kind of a predicament, rescue it (remembering to handle it as little as possible so that it does not stink of humans) and release it in the area in which it was found, during the night when there are few dogs, people and traffic around to threaten it. Only adopt it if it is still there the following morning.

This detailed consideration of fox cubs (which are increasingly common in urban areas) serves to illustrate the advice which can be applied to any apparently abandoned young mammal: do not act on impulse but leave it alone and keep well out of the way. Your very presence is enough to frighten off the parent, and if you should actually touch the baby your human smell could be enough for a parent to abandon the creature permanently, or even to kill it. This applies to all carnivorous species, large and small, and also to deer, rodents and most insectivores.

If you know for certain that the young animal is sick or injured, then you can consider helping but, once again, be realistic about your chances of success and bear in mind all the consequences and the need for substantial commitment. If you know for certain that a lactating mother has been killed, you can consider taking the little one into care (and if you actually find a dead or severely injured lactating mammal, make every effort to find and rescue its young as well). But if it is still with the rest of the litter in its own den, and is old enough not to depend entirely on milk, leave the litter in the den and leave fresh food for them (including drinking water and perhaps some diluted milk) regularly and discreetly, without revealing yourself and preferably without leaving your smell on the food. This will save all the major problems of subsequent rehabilitation. It is a much better system than taking the young out of their wild setting and trying to rear them under artificial conditions.

There is one particular case in which a young mammal definitely will need your help, and that is the autumn hedgehog "orphan". These lone second-litter youngsters have been born too late in the season to be heavy enough for surviving the long winter hibernation, for which they need a minimum weight of 1lb. If they are below weight in November, they will die during the winter and you should try to rescue them from that fate, especially if an underweight juvenile has already collapsed into a dangerously comatose state. Hedgehogs are much easier to care for than most wild animals, and also seem to retain their independence even if they have been in quite close contact with humans. House them indoors (ideally in a garage) in a box with plenty of bedding—dry leaves, sweet hay, crumpled paper, and a hot-water bottle for the very young.

Earlier in the season you should also rescue any little whitish-brown, wobbly hedgehogs if the mother is clearly not going to return to the nest: they will be less than three weeks old, wobbly through hunger and in desperate need of warmth (they will not eat if they are cold) and feeding.

FOSTERING

Try to foster an orphan mammal if possible rather than hand-rear it yourself. Some domestic cats and bitches seem to have a passion for motherhood, quite regardless of the species they are given to foster. A farm bitch will sometimes seek to save the life of a lamb, licking a new-born weakling vigorously to keep its circulation going after a difficult birth, then curling up beside it to keep it warm. By contrast, there was a broody hen who quite aggressively adopted a collie's litter and insisted on brooding the puppies, to their delight, only releasing them for suckling by their bemused mother when the hen decided the moment was right.

Even a guinea-pig will sometimes adopt a fairly similar species like a chinchilla. In most cases it is better to match the species of mother and orphan, and many lactating mothers will accept foster-young slipped in among their own when they are not looking. However, others will kill (and eat) foster-young and possibly do the same with their own offspring because of the disturbance and "contamination"; this is a particular risk with mustelids and lagomorphs. Successful fostering and cross-fostering (that is, different species) depend primarily on the individual temperament of the mother, the way in which an orphan is introduced to the mother and the surroundings in which she is required to receive the adoptee.

Farm livestock are often fostered, especially calves on a nurse cow which readily accepts strangers or can be persuaded to do so during her long nine-month lactation. Sheep are usually more reluctant and have to be tricked into it by disguising the alien lamb's smell. Some sows would readily suckle every piglet in the herd, given the opportunity and whether or not they are themselves in milk, but others are more choosy, especially in intensive situations, though usually they are quick to share piglets in the open. Goat kids are frequently cross-fostered on to ewes, and conversely lambs on to nannies. A mare will accept another mare's foal for up to three or four days after her own foal is born; deer, however, tend to bite or kick the offspring of other deer.

HAND-REARING

The easiest orphans to rear are the domesticated species, already adapted to some degree of human contact. There will be none of the problems of sheer terror that a wild animal experiences, nor the pitfalls of rehabilitation. In addition, much more is known about the needs of domesticated animals including their nutritional needs, their physiology, their behaviour patterns, and the specific effects of a wide range of veterinary treatments. Any veterinary surgeon can tell you how to rear an orphan puppy, kitten or farm animal, and some of that advice can be adapted in caring for similar wild species. For example, if you are caring for a young deer you could apply many of the principles of calf-rearing including the type of accommodation and the methods of giving it milk, but you have to be constantly aware that by hand-feeding it you are probably condemning it to a life of captivity.

ACCOMMODATION

As usual, consider the animal in the wild. Many mammals are born completely defenceless—blind, deaf and barely able to crawl. Most of the carnivores have at least some fur and lagomorphs are well furred (hares fully so) but rodents are virtually naked. Indeed, it can be very difficult to tell one rodent "pinky" from another species, and clearly their major requirement will be warmth, warmth, and more warmth. Even the furry carnivores need extra warmth at first, and all of this group need protection from accidents like predatory raids or falling off high surfaces or, in due course, from wandering away from the "nest". In the wild they are all born and initially reared in dark, secret places, generally underground in burrows, dens, sets, lairs and holes.

Other mammals, however, are like chicks in that they are born ready to get up and go almost the moment they tumble from the womb. All their senses are fully operative; they have a good coat of hair or wool and, after a brief struggle, they master the use of their legs and are able to stagger, then walk and even run within an hour of the birth. They need this ability as a matter of life and death: they are the herbivorous ungulates that will be attacked as prey by the carnivores and they have to be able to escape and run with the herd.

Table II shows how the mammals divide between these broad groupings and gives details about the new-born young of different species.

Carnivores, Insectivores and Rodents

The helpless, immature young of this group need a warm, protected environment and a great deal of early attention. If you find a wild orphan, its priority is warmth, especially if it is a pinky. Normally, young animals in this group would be in a litter with several nest-mates, snuggling together to keep warm, and an orphan on its own will thus be at a considerable disadvantage. If your airing cupboard is unavailable, a hot-water bottle is an instant source of heat and comfort (well padded to avoid direct contact) underneath a snug, draughtproof cardboard box or perhaps a plastic washing-up bowl. Make a good nest of sweet hay, soft tissues or pet-shop bedding so that the animal is completely enveloped: create a hole inside the hay and line it with shredded tissues or perhaps old socks—something soft and warm to cuddle into. The hot-water bottle should be replaced by a more sophisticated heating arrangement as soon as possible but do not overheat animals like leverets, which in the wild are not in enclosed nests, or fox and badger cubs. Make quite sure the nest-box is draughtproof and dry, and try to keep the temperature inside it at a steady level. An electric plant propagator or a clean, dry aquarium are other good containers for pinkies, with built-in heating units, but a cardboard box has the advantage that it can be discarded for a fresh one to avoid a build-up of dirt, disease and parasites. Hygiene is very important, especially for the very young and even more for those that have not had adequate colostrum (first-milk) from their mothers, and bedding and floor litter need to be changed frequently.

TABLE II
NEWBORN MAMMALS

SPECIES	AVERAGE LITTER SIZE	AVERAGE BIRTH WEIGHT (g)	EYES OPEN BY (d = days, w = weeks)	NATURAL WEANING AGE (d = days, w = weeks, m = months)	STATE AT BIRTH
Badger	3	90	10 – 14 d	12-14 w	Sparse fur
Bat	1	–	6 d	6 w	Sparse fur
Cat, domestic	–	–	2 w	6 w	Furred
Cat, wild	4 – 5	–	Birth	4 m	Furred
Cattle	1	–	Birth	9 m	Precocial
Deer	1 – 2	–	Birth	8 – 12 m	Precocial
Dog	–	–	2 w	–	Furred
Dolphin	1	–	Birth	12 – 18 m	Precocial
Dormouse	4	–	18 d	–	Pinky
Ferret	6 – 8	9 – 10	28 d	7 – 8 w	Sparse fur
Fox	4 – 5	100 – 130	8 d	6 w	Furred
Gerbil	4	2.5 – 3.5	21 d	4 w	Pinky
Goat	1 – 2	–	Birth	–	Precocial
Guinea pig	3	70 – 90	Birth	3 – 4 w	Furred
Hamster	6 – 12	2	5 – 7 d	20 – 25 d	Pinky
Hare, Brown	2 – 3	110	Birth	7 d	Furred
Hedgehog	5	11 – 25	13 – 14 d	4 – 6 w	White spines
Mole	3 – 4	3.5	22 d	4 – 5 w	Pinky
Mouse, House	5 – 6	1	7 – 8 d	18 – 21 d	Pinky
Mouse, Wood	5 – 6	1 – 2	16 d	18 – 21 d	Pinky
Otter	2 – 3	–	35 d	10 w	Fine fur
Porpoise	1	8 kg	Birth	–	–
Rabbit	3 – 7	30 – 40	7 – 10 d	3 – 7 w	Some fur
Rat	6 – 10	5	6 – 14 d	3 – 4 w	Pinky
Seal, Common	1	9 – 11 kg	Birth	4 – 6 w	Precocial
Seal, Grey	1	14.5 kg	Birth	17 d	Long white coat
Shrew, Common	5 – 7	0.5	18 – 21 d	22 d	Pinky
Shrew, Water	3 – 8	1	22 d	27 – 37 d	Pinky
Squirrel, Grey	5 – 6	13 – 17	4 – 5 w	8 – 10 w	Pinky
Squirrel, Red	3	10 – 15	28 – 32 d	8 – 10 w	Pinky
Stoat	9	–	5 – 6 w	7 – 12 w	Fine white fur
Vole, Bank	4	2	12 d	18 d	Pinky
Vole, Water	4 – 6	7.5 – 10	8 d	14 d	Pinky
Whale, Blue	1	2,500 kg	Birth	6 – 7 m	Precocial
Whale, Pilot	1	—	Birth	Up to 22 m	Precocial

The next stage will be a "nursery" as the young begin to open their eyes and become more active and exploratory. Plan it so that the original heated nest-box is still available if they choose to use it but offer another sleeping area away from the heat so that you can judge when the heat is no longer necessary. Many animals begin to climb at this stage, or sneak through little gaps, so beware. Otherwise, encourage activity and play by furnishing the nursery with perhaps branches to climb on and corners to hide in, depending on the species.

Young squirrels soon need to be caged and they might as well start off in a cage, with a tall box inside as a drey. Fox and badger cubs need an artificial earth as a dark place to hide in: give them a tea-chest on its side or, preferably, a box with its own sliding door. The box needs to be big enough to accommodate the animal right up to the time of its release and it need this "permanent" bolt hole in order to feel secure. The box will also be the means of transporting the animal to its release site, where it can be left as a temporary shelter while the animal gets used to its surroundings.

When a wild animal reaches the weaning stage it is probably ready to be moved outside into rehabilitation quarters (described in Chapter 9). Make sure it is properly acclimatised first and no longer needs or receives supplementary heating, but do try and move it outside into more elaborate quarters as soon as possible, especially if it is going to be rehabilitated. Cubs (which should not be kept in the house at all for preference and certainly not after they are three or four weeks old, when they no longer need supplementary heating) will do well in a nursery in, say, a garage or outhouse within a cage, kennel or big rabbit or ferret hutch with lots of bedding, but they should not be indoors at all from the age of six weeks, when they will need much more space, preferably in a fox-proof outdoor run or at least with the full freedom of a shed or outhouse. If the animal is to make a successful return to the wild, the sooner it is ready for release, the better, depending of course on the season as well as its own state of health and independence. The question of timing of release is also discussed in Chapter 9.

Bats, which have such different habits to other animals, have special accommodation requirements. If you find a baby bat which does prove to be an orphan, it will need to be kept warm at all times in a special cage designed so that it can hang from its toes upside down in customary bat fashion: use the type of cage described for adult bat casualties, with grippable surfaces on roof and walls, and give it a strip of fur as a substitute mother to snuggle into (even an adult bat would appreciate this). When the time is right, encourage it to fly in a securely closed room (with no cat or dog hiding under the table) so that it can become a proficient flier with properly developed muscles. However, hand-reared juvenile bats will probably remain dependent on you for life: it is almost impossible to teach them how to catch and manipulate prey, and many will actually be terrified of flying insects!

Livestock and Deer

The larger herbivores have simpler accommodation needs in that artificial heat is not usually needed, but of course they do require more space: you can hardly fit a fawn into a cardboard box in the living room. However, you will need to keep young deer indoors at first, or at least confined in a loose-box. If you do try and rear a young deer, it is almost inevitable that it will never be returned to the wild unless it is one of a group or at least a pair of young. If its only contact is with humans, its imprinting will be too strong for it to be rehabilitated.

It would be nice if young deer could be accommodated in a grassed pen with very high wire netting and an open-fronted shelter where they can come for their milk but this idea is unworkable. For a start, they will be terrified of you and will not only dash away from you, never to discover what a milk bottle is, but will also probably injure themselves on the pen netting by hurling against it in an attempt to escape.

A young deer would be better in a straw-littered loose-box so that it can get used to you and your milk bottle. It also needs heat if it is very young and in due course it requires access to soil, which it will eat (perhaps for minerals) and you can either put a bowl of soil in the stall or offer fresh turves every now and then. Save the outdoor pen for later.

Domestic livestock are much simpler and if *you* cannot cope with orphans someone else can. An orphaned or rejected lamb will be in need of warmth and many a farmer has brought a lamb into the kitchen and kept it next to the Aga. I have met several house-trained lambs who were hand-reared and think of themselves as a member of the family, freely wandering in and out of the house, taking the warmest place by the stove (to the digust of the dog) and even curling up on an old sofa by the fire. They are also the ones who always escape from the field first and prove to be the most awkward to herd: they have no fear of humans and often very little respect for familiar dogs. Incidentally, do make quite sure that an orphan of a wild species is never allowed to become familiar with your dog if it is to be rehabilitated, because it will prance up to the first dog it meets in the wild, with disastrous results.

Normally, hand-reared livestock are not house pets but are kept in well-ventilated, draught-free loose-boxes on straw bedding. The very young need "igloos" of straw bales where they can lie snugly hidden, though lambs are not a lying-up species and would be much happier in a group. The main reason for housing is really more for your convenience than for the animals' health: it is easier to feed them under cover than out in a field, though except in winter or in very wet and windy weather they will soon be quite happy out in the open with access to a rough, roofed shelter when they feel like it, as long as they have adequate company. Indeed they will probably remain much healthier outside than in: housed animals are subjected to all sorts of viral and bacterial infections, many of them debilitating and some of them fatal.

TABLE III
MILK COMPOSITION FOR DIFFERENT SPECIES

SPECIES	% SOLIDS	COMPOSITION OF SOLIDS CONTENT			ENERGY
		% FAT	% PROTEIN	% CARBO-HYDRATES	Kcal/ml
Cat	27.0	28	40	27	1.74
Cow, Friesian	12.4	26	26	39	0.71
Deer, Fallow	19.6	43	35	17	1.30
Deer, Red	19.6	39	36	19	1.26
Deer, Roe	24.0	50	29	15	1.56
Dog	22.0	50	35	15	1.58
Dolphin, Bottle-nosed	43.0	78	16	3	3.48
Donkey	8.5	7	16	72	0.38
Ferret	23.5	34	25	–	–
Fox	18.1	32	35	25	1.10
Goat	13.0	35	25	35	0.71
Hare	32.2	46	31	5	2.01
Hedgehog	20.6	47	33	9	1.42
Horse	10.9	15	20	59	–
Human	12.6	17	30	50	–
Mink	21.7	33	26	21	1.17
Mouse, House	29.3	50	34	11	1.84
Pig	15.4	41	31	22	–
Polecat	23.5	43	32	20	1.23
Rabbit	31.2	49	32	6	2.06
Reindeer	26.3	41	34	13	1.68
Seal, Grey	67.7	79	17	4	5.66
Sheep	18.2	39	23	27	1.10
Shrew, Greater white-toothed	51.2	62	19	–	3.50
Shrew, Water	35.0	63	31	3	2.42
Squirrel, Grey	39.6	67	20	10	2.85
Wallaby	13.0	33	29	32	0.83
Whale, Blue	57.0	76	19	2	4.58

FEEDING MILK

Milk Composition

One of the major problems in hand-rearing mammals is that every species produces its own special milk, perfectly suited to its own young, and there can be huge differences in the composition of the milks of different species (and even of different types or breeds within a species). The result is that young fed on an inappropriately constituted milk will at the least suffer digestive upset and undernourishment and at worst will die. It may come as a surprise to learn that most mammals, other than calves, are allergic to that staple food, cow's milk, though many find the milk of sheep and especially of goats more acceptable. If you are going to make a habit of hand-rearing orphans, get a backyard goat or stock your freezer with frozen goat's milk and goat's colostrum.

There has been a great deal of research into mammalian milks and Table III shows the composition of the milks of several species. It is by no means comprehensive but will give some guidance about what your orphan might need and which other mammal's milk is nearest to its own mother's, especially in terms of protein and fat content. A large zoo should be able to give advice on milks and how to feed them.

TABLE IV
MILK REPLACERS

Product	% Fat	% Protein	% Carbo-hydrates	Manufacturers
Cimicat	22	34	34	Hoechst
Denkapup	22	24	46	Denkavit
Esbilac	43	34	15	Pet-Ag
Faramate	14	22	56	Volac
Gold Cap SMA	28	12	56	Wyeth
Horsepower	12	24	53	Championship
KMR	26	43	22	Pet-Ag
Lactol	27	24	33	Shirley's
Lamlac	30	25	35	Volac
Litterlac	30	25	35	Volac
Multi-Milk	30	55	–	Pet-Ag
Primilac	25	20	51	Bioserve
Volac Easy-Mix	20	25	40	Volac
Welpi	18+	27+	41	Hoechst

Table IV gives some of the commercial milk replacers or substitutes which are widely used for orphans, with varying degrees of success. These are usually sold in powdered form so that they can be stored for quite long periods and reconstituted with water when the need for milk arises. It is essential that they are properly measured and very carefully mixed. They must be prepared afresh for each feed. The formula can be enriched if necessary: add egg yolk, pure butterfat or animal tallow for extra fat. The temperature of the mixture (or of normal milk) at and throughout each feeding must be correct and consistent too. Some species develop allergies to certain milk substitutes as well as to natural milks. For example, badger cubs often begin to lose facial hair when fed on cow's milk or on Lactol, though the hair will grow again later, and it might be necessary to change to goat's milk or a milk-free soya-based formula. You need to experiment to find the best substance for an individual orphan. Some of the hair-loss problems can be avoided if you make a point of wiping all traces of milk or feed from the animal's muzzle.

However, one vital substance is very difficult to reproduce in the laboratory or factory, and that is **colostrum**. Colostrum is a nourishing, easily-digested milk produced by several species immediately after birth to give condensed nutrients to the newly born mammal and above all to give it essential antibodies without which it will probably die or at least be susceptible to every possible infection in the new, non-sterile world it has just entered. Without those colostrum antibodies, the survival of most mammal species is very much at stake, and even if the nutritional elements of colostrum can be supplied, the antibodies remain elusive, especially as they are also absorbed by close contact with the natural mother.

If you do not have a frozen store of goat's or cow's colostrum, try the following mixture to compensate for the nutrition of colostrum, though it will not help with immunity: one raw egg; half a pint of water; one pint goat's milk; half a teaspoonful of castor oil (if no diarrhoea).

Equipment

Any mammal is at risk the moment it is removed from its natural mother, and that risk is greatly increased by lack of hygiene in its environment, especially in connection with its feeding equipment. Everything you use for feeding an orphan must be scrupulously clean and sterilised every time with something like Milton. Do not lengthen the already long odds against the orphan's survival by neglecting hygiene, however pressed you are for time.

The type of feeding utensil depends on the size of animal and on personal preference. Many people use bottles with teats and you could use calf or lamb teats from agricultural suppliers, human baby teats, puppy and kitten teats, or even doll's teats from a toy shop. The teat hole can be made bigger if necessary to increase the rate of flow.

For mammals from the size of cubs downwards, you could use a plastic syringe, with a short piece of rubber tube rather than a needle at its nozzle. This equipment shows you exactly how much milk the animal has taken, and you can adjust the rate of flow by adjusting the rate at which you ease the plunger—which should be very slowly. For very tiny babies some people use an eye dropper but that is not always easy to control. In an emergency, soak a very clean piece of cloth in the milk and let the orphan suck the cloth.

Feeding Methods

For the first first feed, when you and the orphan are not yet in accord with each other, do not give milk in case it is accidentally inhaled, which is a sure way to induce pneumonia. Instead, give a glucose solution or an electrolyte mix like Lectade until you are both used to the feeding system. Sit on the floor and hold a small animal in your hand, preferably upright or leaning slightly forward in a natural suckling position, or perhaps lying back a little if you feed it carefully (experiment to see which position suits you both). If it is wriggling, wrap a soft cloth or towel around it, but otherwise simply hold it with its back against your palm and with your thumb acting as a surface for it to "tread" against in the way it would naturally paddle against its mother when feeding. Gently work the tip of the teat or soft rubber tubing into its mouth, between the roof and tongue, and very slowly squeeze in a small measure of milk—only as much as it can take in one swallow (see Fig. 42 on p. 136). It might help if you have a drop of milk on the end of the tube to moisten the animal's lips: with luck it will respond to the milk and open its mouth to suck. You might find it easier to ease the tube into its mouth at the corner rather than from the front but take great care not to force the milk down its throat and choke it.

Many people let the animal decide when enough is enough, on the assumption that it will stop accepting milk when its needs are satisfied, but this is a dangerous practice if you are not experienced. You should stop too soon rather than too late, and never give it so much milk that its belly becomes a tight balloon. With many species, it is the output of the mother that limits the ration, not the infant's appetite. Excessive milk will soon lead to digestive upsets as well as making the animal too fat, and if it begins to scour (diarrhoea) it is either receiving too much milk or the milk is too rich, and you should immediately substitute a feed or two of glucose solution and then give a more diluted milk feed, gradually building back to an acceptable strength. If you feed to the point when the milk remains in the animal's mouth and begins to dribble out, you have reached the absolute limit of its capacity and should have stopped sooner.

The frequency of feeding is really rather an arbitrary factor and it is not necessarily appropriate to be guided by wild habits (for example, a hare would only suckle once in twenty-four hours). Most people would feed tiny creatures every two hours, and some would continue that regime night and day, at least for the first two nights. However, if you cannot get any sleep, you will not be much use to the baby! The list below suggests feeding intervals, utensils and possible milks for different species but should only be taken as a guide: each animal is an individual and you should be sensitive to its needs and its behaviour. For all except the horse family, lagomorphs and marine mammals, choose from goat's or ewe's milk, Lactol, Lamlac, Esbilac or a dog or cat milk replacer (Welpi, Litterlac, Cimicat, KMR etc.).

Badgers　Use something like a Catac foster-feeding bottle (kits are usually obtainable from pet shops) with a narrow, supple teat. Slightly enlarge the hole: badger cubs quickly become disheartened if they have difficulty in drawing out the milk. Try Lactol (1 part to 4 parts water at first) but many badgers are allergic. Feed every two hours at first, reducing gradually to five times a day. Increase strength of mixture to 1:3 after the second week, and to 1:2 by the eighth week.

Bats　Use eye-dropper or pipette and feed skimmed milk—not too creamy. Try goat's or ewe's milk. Bats must be kept warm or will not feed.

Deer　Use baby's bottle, calf feeding bottle or lamb bar, and try giving goat's milk or Lamlac—perhaps adding dextrose, cod-liver oil and eggs.

Fox　Avoid cow's milk. Try goat's or Lactol. Feed every three to four hours if small. Bottle-feeding is necessary if cubs are less than four weeks old (chocolate-brown fur, weight about 4-20 oz). Start with syringe feed, graduate to Catac or other pet-shop bottle with teat at two to three weeks. Feed three or four times a day by the age of three to four weeks. Start giving solids at four weeks. Weight at six weeks should be about 36 oz.

Hedgehog　Give colostrum (goat's if necessary) for first 48 hours, then milk and water with glucose or try Complan. If eyes still closed, feed every two to three hours between 7 a.m. and 11 p.m., about 3 ml a feed. If eyes open, feed every three to four hours, 5 ml.

Livestock　Use own species' milk for preference—bottle-fed, or lamb-bar/calfeteria cold-milk systems (can cause digestive upset at first), or bucket-feeding after training. Many appropriate milk substitutes are available.

Otter　This is one for a specialist, who will probably feed the cub on a liquidised mixture based on white fish and Lactol.

Pinkies   It can be very difficult to identify the species in the case of pinkies but most of them flourish on goat's milk. You will need an eye-dropper or pipette, or for slightly bigger ones you could try a doll's feeding bottle.

Rabbits and hares   Ideally, use high-fat, high-protein, low-sugar replacers such as Esbilac. Otherwise try Lactol, Welpi etc., three or four feeds a day—stop before they are full. In the wild the mother suckles very briefly.

Seal   Avoid lactose—do not use milk from other species. Feed a liquidised fish soup (fish, water, cod-liver oil and a fatty acid supplement) by stomach tube if you are an expert.

Squirrel   Typical pinkies—feed every two hours at first, with little doses. When eyes open, feed every four hours between 7 a.m. and 11 p.m.

Stimulation

Keep the little one clean: wipe all traces of milk from its face and anywhere else it has dribbled, using a moist piece of cottonwool (avoid cloths: use something fresh each time), then dry it carefully with tissues or kitchen paper. You must also pay attention to its other end.

Many new-born suckling mammals have to be stimulated to urinate and defecate until they learn how to do this of their own accord. The natural mother licks the infant's rear end before, during and after suckling, and it is important that you should imitate this stimulation by using a piece of damp cottonwool to tickle or gently wipe the genitals. If you do not, the little creature will suffer from an over-full bladder and soon become ill. Assume that this stimulation is necessary, whatever the species, and continue the practice until you have evidence that the animal can urinate and defecate of its own accord, which might take a couple of days or might be a couple of weeks, according to the species and its circumstances. Most should be stimulated immediately after feeding, but hedgehogs often need the treatment both before and after a meal, and deer need it during rather than after feeding.

Weaning

Once the eyes of an immature mammal open, the young animal will become more active and explorative. Now you can start offering something more solid than milk—perhaps Complan, or soft tinned dogfood, or fresh chopped grass as appropriate to the species. The animal should now be in its nursery and needs a constant supply of clean, fresh drinking water, though this will not be used much while milk is still on the menu.

Put a shallow dish of appropriate food where it can easily be found but well away from the nest or earth. The animal will no doubt trample in it and make a filthy mess but in due course it will discover that the food is edible. Give fresh food at least daily, and remove all traces of stale food regularly, watching out for any tendency to cache a meal in a secret hiding place. (Foxes and mustelids are good at this trick.)

Continue the bottle-feeding in the meantime, gradually reducing the amount and frequency, until you are sure the animal is feeding itself happily and properly. Introduce any new foods gradually and do begin to offer variety, both for interest and to ensure a well-balanced diet. When you are satisfied that it has learned to eat more solid food, then you can breathe a sigh of relief and give your milk bottle its last wash. You can also turn off the artificial heat, especially if the orphan has taken the option of moving away from the source of heat.

If a wild youngster is already close to the weaning stage when you take it in, do your best to avoid handling it. See that it can and will lap some diluted milk with glucose in it and, if so, leave it a dish of the milk, a dish of clean drinking water and a dish of soft food. Do not hand-feed it unless there is no option. It is much better for the orphan's eventual rehabilitation if it has as little direct contact with you as possible.

To wean livestock, including deer, the usual method is to encourage them from an early age to eat good hay, young greens and weaning pellets (they will not need much persuasion) and as soon as they are feeding adequately you can either gradually reduce the amount and frequency of milk or just stop it altogether quite suddenly. Consult a livestock book for guidance.

ORPHAN SEALS

Orphan seal pups need quite different rearing to other mammals. As has been stressed before, their needs are best understood by those with experience of this very special mammal, and even they have only imperfect knowledge. There are perhaps three major problems: imprinting, environment and nutrition.

A young seal pup in its first week of life will follow just about anything that moves in the fond hope of a suckle, bleating piteously if it is hungry. Those moving objects might be people walking along a beach, which is one reason why too many seal "orphans" are picked up: it is assumed that the animal is lost and desperate. The pup is then taken home by concerned people and fed on something like cow's milk, with the result that it rapidly loses condition. At this stage, people look for help.

The seals most likely to be found around British coasts are the common and the grey. The grey is generally the bigger species, especially the males, and the pups weigh on average 32 lb at birth, trebling this in less than three weeks! Common pups, which weigh 20-24 lb at birth, also treble their bodyweight during their longer lactation period of four to six weeks.

This colossal rate of growth (an average gain of 4 lb a day for the grey, for example) is achieved by the transfer of the mother's blubber to her pup in the form of very rich, fatty milk, which increases its fat content as the lactation progresses.

Seal pups are intolerant of lactose, and no one has yet produced a seal-milk substitute. At present the best solution seems to be to put the orphan straight on to a diet of fish "soup" (if it is given whole fish too soon, it will possibly develop diarrhoea) but there is a great danger that this early weaning could result in a dwarf adult. However, if there is no other option, at least the soup will keep the pup alive and can help it to grow to a reasonable weight before it is released.

Quite apart from the problem of the right food, there is the problem of getting it into the seal, and this is where experienced handling is essential. Force-feeding is inevitable and an emaciated pup will need a rehydrating fluid for the first day, with no soup until the second day. A fatty fish is needed as the basis of the soup (it is the nearest you will get to blubber) and liquidised herring seems to be appropriate, fed warm through a flexible 12 inch tube attached to a lamb-feeder syringe. The soup is fed for days two to six, but with effect from day four the volume of the soup is gradually reduced and slivers of fish are added—skinned, boned herring cut into pieces about 2 inches by 1 inch in size—and gradually these slivers are increased so that they are slices rather than slivers. Sprats and shrimps can also form part of the diet.

It can be very difficult at first to persuade the pup to swallow its fish. The knack involves carefully opening its mouth wide enough so that you can put the slivers at the back, past the tongue. However, seals are born with a proper set of teeth and you are very likely to have your finger painfully bitten. The whole performance is bound to be stressful to the seal and you must do all you can to reduce the stress, rather than increase it by protecting your own fingers with mouth wedges.

It is to be hoped that this description will deter you from taking home a seal pup unnecessarily. And you still have not reached the stage of changing the diet to live fish, building up the pup's swimming muscles with controlled exercise in a salt-water pool and then finding a good release site away from irate fishing fleets . . .

CHAPTER NINE

REHABILITATION OF WILDLIFE

The word rehabilitation has been mentioned countless times in this book. Its literal meaning is re-enablement and the dictionary definitions of the word include: to reinstate; to restore to former privileges; to bring back into good condition; to make fit, after disablement or illness, for earning a living or playing a part in the world. That last definition, about playing a part in the world, would seem particularly apt in the context of animal rescue.

The foundation stone of wildlife rehabilitation is a complex aggregate of moral, philosophical and practical issues, but the central consideration must be whether or not we have any right to keep any wild animal captive when there is a chance of it flourishing in the wild. There are arguments for and against giving permanent accommodation to an animal too disabled to survive in the wild: even if you consider the individual, as opposed to the species as a whole, there is still the question of the quality of its life and whether it is better to live in what is essentially a state of deprivation, even if it is one of safety and "comfort". (Imagine yourself living involuntarily as the only human being among a crowd of protective snakes or wolves or spiders: they might have your interests at heart and do their utmost to provide you with the right food and accommodation, but could they ever really understand your needs—including your emotional needs—and could you ever wholly trust their motives?)

The philosophy expressed in this book is that the principal aim of a wildlife rescuer should be to nurse an animal to a state of fitness, physically and behaviourally, for a return to its natural habitat and lifestyle among its own kind—that is, back to the wild. Its life in the wild might not be easy or safe, but it is the very adversities of nature which have shaped the species: it is *designed* for its wild niche.

RECUPERATION

Most of this book has been concerned with the rescue and intensive care of distressed animals. Now comes the time when their lives are no longer in danger, their wounds and bones are healing well, their state of shock has been minimised, and they are well on the road to recovery. From here on, everything needs to be geared to the animals' eventual release.

In most cases the aim is to return an animal to its environment as quickly as possible so that its stay in your care is but a hiccup in its normal existence. There are exceptions to the quick turnover policy: some releases are dictated by the season as much as by the animal's fitness, for example. You cannot release a migrant long after the rest of its species have fled to their seasonal habitats; you cannot release a hibernating species in midwinter; you should be cautious about releasing wildfowl during their moult, when so many become unable to fly. It is of course essential to find out as much as you can about the animal's lifestyle and to act in the light of that knowledge.

Perhaps the most important factors in the recuperation period are the opportunity for the animal to exercise itself and regain its muscular strength and co-ordination, the stimulation of its general interest in life after a time of almost suspended living, and the chance to shake off human influences and any trust it might have developed of the human race as a whole. Not every person it meets in the future will be as compassionate as you are. All these factors need to be borne in mind in planning the accommodation and general care of the animal in this final stage.

ACCOMMODATION

For nearly all species of wildlife and livestock, the recuperation accommodation needs to be out of doors but with access to shelter if the animal wishes to make use of it. In broad terms, that means a secure pen or aviary which is both escape-proof and protected from predators or enemies, with a shelter giving protection from the elements and absolute privacy at the animal's option, and a feeding point where food and water can be provided with minimal human intrusion. In appropriate situations you will also need a means of letting the animal find its own way to freedom when it is ready to go, and this place of exit from the pen can be used as a habitual feeding point to which the animal can return at will until it no longer needs your support.

Birds

A bird which has been confined to a cage for more than a few days needs a chance to exercise its wings and build up its flying muscles before it is released. With small birds, a brief period in a simple aviary will be adequate and will give you a chance to assess that they can fly well enough to survive in the wild. This assessment is obviously essential in the case of a bird which has been treated for wing injuries but there can also be problems which were unsuspected when the bird was caged. Primary feather damage, for example, can seriously distort a bird's ability to control the direction and altitude of its flight and in some cases it will need to be kept in an aviary until it has moulted and grown new feathers. There might also be indirect effects from other injuries which could affect flying.

An aviary should therefore be large enough for you to assess the bird's overall fitness, as well as being suitable for its continuing recuperation, and it should be furnished to give the bird plenty of stimulation and appropriate exercise. It should also let the bird feel the warmth of the sun.

Roosting and perching species need **perches** of varying thicknesses, textures and heights so that they have a choice and so that their feet are properly exercised. For preference use rough branches such as the bird would use in the wild, rather than smooth, uniform dowelling. Give them platforms as well as perches, and give seabirds rockeries and artificial cliffs. Cater for activities like climbing, too: nuthatches would appreciate a tree trunk or two, or pieces of rough bark fixed on vertical surfaces, where nuts and larvae can be hidden. In a more permanent aviary add shrubs and climbing plants for a combination of cover, perching and variety, or introduce split-log plant containers planted with ivy and other instant greenery. Set up a rustic roosting box, which might prove more attractive to the bird if its entrance is camouflaged with rough bark. Have a small part of the aviary roofed with thatch or solid materials for protection from hot sun or heavy rain.

Ground-loving birds like pheasants need plenty of natural cover at ground level and low vantage points as well as a high roost perch. Scatter a few conifer branches, straw bales and wattle hurdles in the pen and give them something like a wooden fence rail or a shed roof from which to view the world. Pheasants enjoy sunbathing on a roof, especially if it is pitched, and that is true for other poultry which do not fly unless they must.

Most birds need shallow **bathing water** as well as drinking water (even owls sometimes bathe, and diurnal raptors might dip either their breast feathers or more likely their food in the bathwater), but ground birds prefer dust-bathing and should have access to a box of dry soil kept under cover, perhaps in a low-roofed area where their grain can also be scattered. A permanent rainwater pond will attract insect life, which is good food for so many birds, and a few clumps of nettles or brambles will also draw in the invertebrates or you could plant hop vines to lure the insects and act as a windbreak as well.

Penned waterfowl, once their plumage is in good enough condition, need a pool at least deep enough for them to get their heads right under water and preferably enough for a splash-bath. The pool must be kept clean (the birds tend to dunk their food in the water and also defecate in it) and should therefore either have a constant self-flushing flow of fresh water through it or be easy to empty and scrub out daily. The area around the pool will quickly become a trampled bog, which is not good for captive birds, and it needs an ample concrete apron. Waterfowl also make a muddy mess around drinking points but the ground can be protected with small-mesh wire netting laid flat so that the birds can stand comfortably and the splashed water can drain away.

The **floor** of an aviary or pen is usually of turf and if it is in constant use it will soon be scratched to bare soil or trampled to mud. (With foresight you can take a tip from ornamental pheasant keepers: lay wire mesh over the soil and let the grass grow through it.) Keep grass reasonably in trim if the birds do not—say, about 4 inches high. Plant with a good mixture of grasses and herbs to supply a variety of fresh green food and to attract insects. In a temporary aviary you could introduce pots of suitable food plants, berried shrubs and hydroponic grasses, all of which will not only provide food but also stimulate the birds to forage and learn not to depend on their food bowl. Waterfowl pens need shrubbery as cover for the birds and also a very rough shelter of some kind for optional use: even ducks do not enjoy torrential rain, and all birds dislike strong wind.

The **fencing** of an aviary is installed on the same principles as that for penning waterfowl or some of the mammals. The aim is both to keep your recuperants in and to keep food-stealers and predators out. Use welded wire mesh for preference: it is much stronger and more rigid than hexagonal chicken-wire. Make the fence at least 6 feet high above ground level and add a strip of smaller diameter mesh to at least 2 feet high from the base and buried another foot or two into and under the ground to deter diggers, whether they are predators and scavengers trying to get in or birds trying to get out (some ground birds do try and dig to freedom). The buried mesh should form an L-shape as a further line of defence against external diggers (see Fig. 44). For ground birds, put some cladding at the bottom of the pen sides to act as a windbreak and to give them privacy.

For most birds, **roof** the aviary with mesh, which also keeps out unwanted wild birds, but this can be expensive for larger areas. Some people therefore use soft netting but you should beware of snow: a heavy snowfall will sag such a roof badly and could bring the whole lot down. The roof should also be designed to keep out raiding cats and foxes, both of which are good climbers and jumpers, and they can be further deterred by turning out the top foot or two of the vertical mesh at an angle of 45 degrees, or you can run several strands of barbed-wire on jibs at a similar angle.

Birds of prey need their own aviaries: do not place them so that they terrorise other species merely by their presence and shape and do not have them in pens adjacent to other birds of prey unless there is something solid between them, or there could be some fights. However, the care of birds of prey is really not for amateurs. For a start, you need a licence to keep a diurnal raptor in captivity for more than a few days, even if it is injured. In addition, a good falconer has an important role to play in the rehabilitation of birds of prey, which really need to be "hacked back", that is, gradually acclimatised for the wild by standard falconry techniques which exercise the bird and build up its strength, getting its "eye" in for hunting again. Finally, the birds should only be released from their recuperation aviary direct, rather than taken elsewhere for release, and it is therefore essential that the immediate environment is suitable and appropriate territory for the bird when it is freed.

If you are accommodating birds of prey, they do not require a screened area behind which they can retire for privacy—and they will do so whenever they see a human. This screened platform or box should perhaps be at your shoulder level but with ample head room and landing approach. They also need some stout perching branches of varying thickness to keep their feet in good order and many also like to stand on top of posts or tall stumps. Most important of all, they need a high feeding station designed so that you need never invade their territory and also so that they can continue to use the same station when they have been released. The platform should therefore extend outside the aviary and have a hatch through which you can deposit the food and also free the birds in due course (see Fig. 45). Owls will appreciate a landing post outside the aviary a few yards from the feeding station and close to copse-type cover if possible, so that they can assess the situation before they fly in to feed.

Until you are experienced, please take owls and day-flying raptors to the licensed specialists for care and release, or at least consult the Hawk Trust's new National Centre for Owl Conservation in Norfolk, breed-and-release schemes like BOBARS (British Owl Breeding And Release Scheme), or a local owl rescuer or falconer, but be a little wary of those whose interest might be more in keeping birds to breed from them for profit than in rehabilitating them in the wild.

Mammals

The smaller mammals are easily housed in hutches, chicken arks etc. and will probably need very little acclimatistion before release. A long-stay **hedgehog,** however, needs a proper run with the base of the wire mesh buried vertically

FIG. 43 CONVALESCENT DEN FOR BADGERS AND FOXES

Tea-chest in shed, with hinged inspection lid. Open end is facing wall, with small gap between wall and chest just big enough for animal's access. Entrance protected from direct light and draughts and hidden from view.

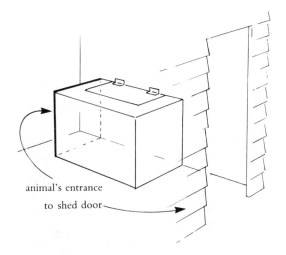

animal's entrance

to shed door

FIG. 44   OUTDOOR AVIARY AND PEN NETTING

Designed to keep diggers and climbers on right side of wire. Main netting should be about 6 feet above ground level—rigid welded mesh rather than hexagonal chickenwire. Use smaller mesh size on lowest section to deter entry by predators. Smaller-mesh footings should be turned horizontally under turf to deter diggers, whilst anti-climber overhangs should be at 45 or 90° with appropriate supports.

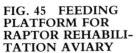

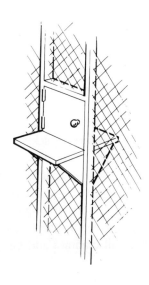

FIG. 45   FEEDING PLATFORM FOR RAPTOR REHABILI-TATION AVIARY

Hatch door allows feeding from outside and can also be left open for post-release feeding.

for a few inches, and it will appreciate a chance to explore its environment. It is not going to move with any great speed and should be quite easy to supervise on its garden strolls.

The **smaller mustelids** can move like lightning and are expert escapologists, though a good ferret hutch should be adequate for their recuperation period if it has direct access to a securely fenced run with very small mesh size and a wire roof (see Fig. 39 on p. 128). It is essential that they have somewhere dark and private to sleep and also protection from hot sun as some of them quickly succumb to heatstroke. Put them in a shady place (remembering that the sun moves round) or paint a hutch or shed roof white to reflect away the sun's rays, and paint the inside of a hutch white, too, so that you are reminded to keep it clean.

Give **all small mammals** an interesting environment, even in the short term: provide trenches and drainpipes for mustelids to explore, or give hedgehogs plenty of dead leaves to nose around in. Always supply fresh drinking water. The mustelids are very clean in their toilet habits and will choose one corner of their hutch or run, which makes cleaning up after them much simpler.

Squirrels can live in an aviary if the mesh is tough enough to resist their formidable rodent teeth—try chainlink or rigid welded mesh. Give them lots of climbing surfaces and places to jump to and from: branches, tree trunks, wooden posts, or even a child's small climbing frame! Fix up a simple wooden drey and provide bedding material for the squirrel to busy itself with: do not deprive it of useful activity by making the bed for it. Squirrels are very busy animals, even in winter. But if a squirrel *is* active, it is no doubt ready for release and needs to be free. However, grey squirrels are legally classed as vermin and technically you are not allowed to release them again into the wild: consult your local NCC office. Red squirrels, conversely, are a carefully protected species in Britain (in fact you need an NCC licence to keep one at all, even for first aid treatment) and should be released where they were living originally.

Bats are special. They need a properly designed bat cage so that they hang upside down in peace and they need plenty of warmth right through their treatment and convalescence to speed their recuperation (34-36 °C). They also recover more quickly and feed better if handled frequently, which is quite the opposite to most wild patients.

It is important that a bat has ample flying practice before it is released: it must be able to fly strongly. Encourage flying at mealtimes in a secure room with ample soft landings (cushions etc.) until it has regained its skills and strength. Keep a sharp watch on where it chooses to land: bats can hide in very small crannies and be difficult to find. Do not try and catch a bat in flight because you will probably damage its wing and have to start nursing it all over again. Wait for it to settle and then pick it up.

It is essential to help a bat recover in the shortest possible time if it is to be rehabilitated—twenty days at the very most from the time you bring it in. If you have kept a bat too long for rehabilitation, it will have to remain in captivity for the rest of its life—and that could be many years. They actually make much loved pets but do be aware of the legal situation: the law seeks to protect all bats.

Foxes and badgers are much more of a problem in all respects. To begin with, their recuperation period might be a matter of months, especially if they are orphans being prepared for the wild. Next, there is the question of where they are to be released. Like birds of prey, the ideal site for the recuperation pen is adjacent to the release area so that they can return for self-help feeding at will and perhaps find security as well. However, both species are strongly territorial and the release site must be carefully chosen. It might be necessary to transport them to a release site elsewhere but this should only be done under expert advice and supervision. It is important that the animal is allowed to become familiar with the local area while it still has an option to return "home" to its old quarters if necessary.

Then there is the problem that they might make strenuous and determined efforts to escape before you want them to leave. Fox cubs, for example, get very excited about August, which is the natural dispersal time for a wild litter, and are capable of clambering over a 6-foot fence at that stage. Adult badgers are often quite desperate to escape from captivity. Indeed, both species become depressed and neurotic in close confinement and their pens must not be mean. In the wild they range extensively; they like to explore, to forage, to mark their boundaries and to dig new dens. Even a reared orphan has these urges. It can be kept in a secure outhouse for the first few weeks of its life but by the age of about six weeks it will long to explore the world beyond its den. It is also the age at which they can become too boisterous for the humans who had found them sweet and cuddly as babies, and you need to be especially careful with a growing young badger who, in its rough-and-tumble games, will forget that you are not a badger and could give you a bite to remember. When the young have reached this stage, they should be given every opportunity to explore: start them off in a pen with direct access from the shed until they are ready to be given a free choice through an ever-open gate to the outside world.

Pens for foxes and badgers of any age need careful design and building. It will take ingenuity and quite a lot of money to create an escape-proof and properly furnished pen. The perimeter fencing is similar to that of a waterfowl pen, described earlier, but the chainlink or welded mesh needs to be of a heavier gauge so that it can defy a determined badger's powerful jaws. You would be wise to pay attention to the animals' considerable digging abilities: their point of attack for the freedom dig will inevitably be where the fencing meets the ground and you should reverse the pattern of bird pens by having the buried horizontal section running *inwards* in the pen, with the overhang at the top of the fence also turning inwards to fool a climbing fox (see Fig. 44). However, a badger in particular should be allowed to express its urge to dig within the pen and create its own complex tunnel system—as long as those tunnels do not end up on the wrong side of the wire by mistake. For a permanent resident it is worth using concrete along the whole length of the perimeter as an anti-digging barrier. An adult fox, incidentally, can find its way through a hole 4 inches square.

If the pen is also a release pen, it needs a two-way exit by which you can control the animal's comings and goings. Any gate you use yourself must be a double-gate system to avoid the risk of an animal bolting for freedom as you enter or leave the pen.

If a shed is not an integral part of the pen, you must provide an artificial sett or earth. Ideally this should include the animal's original box, adequately weatherproofed and familiar, or otherwise devise a dark, dry and completely private den, preferably underground for better insulation, but make it with an inspection hatch for emergencies (the most popular basis is a large diameter concrete pipe). Best of all is something that can also serve as a transporter if the animal is to be released elsewhere: the simplest way to catch it for transporting is to let it enter the security of the den in its own time, shut it in and pick up the whole contraption so that it travels in a familiar environment.

In theory, foxes like a higher arch to their earth entrance whereas badgers like a flatter semicircle more suited to their own ground-hugging shape, but size is more important than shape, and more important still is that the opening should be positioned so that approaching people (or dogs) outside the pen are not visible to the animal in the den (a dog-leg opening is ideal).

Let the animal have access to plenty of clean hay and straw so that it can make its own bed within the den. Badgers make quite a business of bedmaking, and they "air the sheets" every now and then by dragging all the litter outside to dry and freshen.

A barren environment is as soul-destroying for badgers and foxes as for humans. A good pen contains growing trees and shrubs, rough bramble and nettle patches, or at the very least tree trunks to climb on and dig under, straw bale "houses" to hide in or behind and, in the case of lonely orphans, plenty of toys to play with, chew, worry, "fight" and "kill". At that stage the orphans needs to be denied direct contact with people (or with dogs) and therefore needs substitute playthings. Like puppies and children, they can become very attached to a particular soft toy or piece of blanket, if it can stand their attentions.

Otters are cousins of the badger (both are mustelids) and a captive otter's pen is broadly similar, with the addition of a swimming pool. However, it is unlikely that you will look after an adult otter (and definitely inadvisable), it being preferable for orphans to be raised by specialists like the Otter Trust in Suffolk.

In the unlikely event that you will be accommodating a **seal,** the problem will be to give the animal adequate exercise for its swimming muscles. Orphans in particular need to develop these and can be given access to an appropriately deep pool from three to four weeks old. They also need to learn the art of catching *live* fish during the following month or two and should not be released until they are proficient at both fishing and swimming.

The rehabilitation of **deer** is a delicate business. If you are dealing with an adult, it should have been in an outdoor pen or paddock right from the start and should remain in the same pen until it is due for direct release. Deer-proof fencing has to be at least 6 feet high for a fit deer, though farmed species can be taught to respect an electric livestock fence. The land should be free-draining and the deer will appreciate plenty of natural hiding places—contours providing hills and hollows, or thickets, and trees for shade. An open-fronted lean-to shed is excellent housing but usually unnecessary, and deer also like a wallow if you can arrange this. You really need a paddock situated near suitably safe open land and woodland because release, whether planned or stolen by the deer, can only be by opening the gates and letting the animal walk out of its own accord in its own time. To try and transport it elsewhere could kill it.

A young deer does well in a roomy but draughtproof building leading to an exercise yard or pen. Exercise is important to a growing animal and if it is a member of a herd species (red and fallow) it also needs the company of its own kind as it matures. Never keep one of these on their own as adults.

Amphibians and Reptiles

The needs of reptiles like **snakes and lizards** are relatively simple—peace, water and warmth. They should be kept in a roomy and well-furnished dry container such as an aquarium or smooth-sided box, at a constant ambient temperature suitable to their habitats. Provide a water bowl big enough for the snake to curl into. Temperate species do better in outdoor reptiliaries unless they are hibernating. Land **tortoises** need a dry environment; they are of course very slow movers but can plod with determination for quite long distances so that out of doors they need confinement in a pen unless your garden is escape-proof. **Turtles** or **terrapins** need a swimming pond with very clean water and will be best in an aquarium but must have a dry island when they want to leave the water—otherwise they will probably die of exhaustion.

An old aquarium is also suitable for **amphibians** (frogs, toads and newts) but they need a moist atmosphere and access to shallow bathing water, with a dry standing area as well. Frogs hop—their accommodation needs a lid—but toads merely crawl. In winter various reptiles and amphibians need different conditions in their hibernation quarters, though some of the tropical species should not be allowed to hibernate. Read John Cooper's *Manual of Exotic Pets* for details of vivariums for long-term exotic reptile and amphibian patients, including temperature control, floor materials and "furniture".

ASSESSMENT

If a casualty has been in your care for more than a few days, your assessment of its fitness for release has to be much more thorough than a general impression that it is "better". Here are some of the factors you need to consider, whatever the species, bearing in mind that these factors have to be set in the context of its wild environment rather than confinement. Are its abilities adequate for the wild?

Physical Abilities

- Has its original problem been properly diagnosed and adequately treated? The bones of many wild animals often heal better than you might expect. As long as the vet says the casualty is well on the way, it is probably better to release it than to keep it longer and risk the development of disease or of behavioural and long-term nutritional problems.
- Is it mobile? Can it move well enough to get its food, escape its enemies and protect itself? Is it able to rest properly? (For example, will roosting be difficult if a bird's leg is disabled?)
- What about its senses? Can it see, smell and hear well enough to find food and recognise danger? Does it have any sign of eye or ear disease? Have you tested its visual and aural reactions? If it is a raptor, did it become an RTA originally because its eyesight was defective?
- Are a bird's feathers in good condition? Are they spotlessly free of oil and detergent? Are they waterproof? Has a young chick grown its proper

feathers to replace the down? What about a bird's flight feathers: are they strong and complete? Is it beyond the moult and therefore in generally good feather?

● Does it have adequate plumage for display and other social behaviour?
● Is it plump enough to withstand the imminent winter, or strong enough to make a migratory journey? Are its teeth/beak/claws adequate for all purposes? Is it alert enough to be safe?

Behaviour

● Is it humanised or imprinted on another species? Will it be able to relate to its own species?
● Is it too tame for its own good? Will it quickly fall victim to people or dogs or, on the other hand, is it so unafraid of people that it could be a danger to them? (Hand-reared male deer, for example, should never be released in the wild: they are more than likely to attack people, especially in the rut.)

Disease

● Is the animal still reasonably resistant to the diseases it will encounter in the wild?
● Has it come to you in order to escape an epidemic in its own area (for example, seal virus) and is that epidemic still a threat?
● Is a hand-reared animal adequately immunised? Has a badger or fox been vaccinated against leptospirosis or parvovirus? Is a de-parasited animal *too* "clean" and therefore vulnerable in the wild?
● Will the animal introduce a disease into the wild, either because it has been transferred from a different area where different diseases are prevalent (for example, tuberculosis and myxomatosis) or because it is carrying a domestic disease acquired from its contact with humans, livestock and pets during its confinement?

The Law

● Is it legal to release the species in the wild?
● Was it legal to confine it in the first place?

IDENTIFICATION

It could be of more than passing interest if the animal can be labelled in some way before release. For one thing, you need to know whether or not it manages to survive in the wild. Has your treatment of its problems been successful in the long term? Was your assessment of its fitness adequate? What can you learn if not? It is no good devoting all that time and compassion to a patient and then casting it back into the wild with no idea of whether or not you did the right things. Was it perhaps your fault that it subsequently died? However close you have been to an animal, do not expect to be able to recognise it later: mark it in some way so that you know for sure which it is and keep your own detailed records of your marking system, with a note of all the circumstances relating to the animal's original rescue and its release.

Another important reason for marking is to help naturalists, conservationists and others with an interest in wildlife and ecology to monitor a species in its environment, in the hope that a greater understanding will lead to a more secure future for the species.

Mammals can often be marked with a tattoo, especially if they are already under sedation for other purposes in the veterinary surgery. Typical areas for tattooing are the ears or the inner thigh, though seals are generally identified by a tag under the arm-pit. Talk to the Mammal Society about methods of identification: people have used all manner of ingenious devices. But beware of anything involving a collar, which can so easily get caught up and trap or throttle the animal.

Birds can also be tattooed, under the wing, and the markings should last for years. Your vet can show you how to do it. However, the most common method of identifying birds is by leg-rings, and the numbering system works on a national basis so that the whole business is unified and co-ordinated. The major ringing scheme in this country is administered by the British Trust for Ornithology (BTO) but the ringing committee has strict criteria regarding who can ring a bird and what species are ringed. Do not even think of ringing a bird yourself unless you are experienced: a ring of the wrong size, or fitted at the wrong time, can either constrict the bird's leg dangerously in due course or, if too loose, will get caught up, and anway you must have a ringing licence. Advice on the fairly complicated subject of birds which *must* be ringed *as soon as they are taken into captivity* can be found in Chapter 10.

It is common practice for a licensed ringer to be asked to go to a rehabilitation centre and ring several birds at once as long as the centre can guarantee to provide accurate information on when and where each bird is subsequently released. For the name of your nearest ringer, contact the BTO. There are other ringing schemes, too—for example that of the British Bird Council (BBC).

A Licensed Rehabilitation Keeper (LRK) licence allows certain people who have the facilities, experience and expertise to tend birds and successfully release them back to the wild (this rehabilitation is essential to the licence) and to keep for up to six weeks certain species of disabled birds which would normally have to be registered with the Department of the Environment and ringed. The fees payable for licences and registrations are high. You might find that your vet is an LRK, and as long as the bird's treatment is under his instruction and supervision your problems might be solved.

THE RELEASE SITE

Selection of a release site is the culmination of all your efforts to rescue a wild creature and it can also be the ruin of them. You need to assess the site as intelligently and thoroughly as you originally assessed your patient's predicament and needs. You do not want to have subjected it to all that stress for nothing. The most important aspects to consider are the following:

- Is the habitat capable of maintaining an animal of this species and does it already do so? If it does not, why not?
- Can the area supply the type and quantity of food and water needed?
- Does it offer the necessary shelter, cover and security? Will it give reasonable safety from hunters, poachers, vandals, drivers and other human predators? Will the landowner and neighbouring property owners welcome or at least accept the animal's presence? Will the animal be a nuisance or danger to people living in the area?
- Is there any threat (now or in the future) that the site might be contaminated in any way, for example, by oil, chemicals, poisons or other pollution, or suffer from flooding, large-scale forestry clearance or other major habitat destruction?
- Are there sufficient reasonably safe routes out of the area if the animal wishes to leave it? Think of useful "highways" like hedgerows and streams, and think of danger zones like motorways and high-voltage electricity cables. Always think of an environment in three dimensions and as part of a wider area, never in isolation. Are there other suitable habitats linked by these routes so that the animal has freedom of choice?
- Is the animal of a territorial species and, if so, is the release site already the territory of another animal or group? Will an existing social group accept the animal or will it be attacked or ostracised? Does the site offer the animal an opportunity to breed and rear young?
- Is the animal already familiar with the area? If so, the animal will know where to find food, where to hide, what hazards to avoid—unless the habitat, food sources or local social structures have changed during too long an absence.

● Is the site reasonably accessible so that you can keep a discreet eye on the animal's progress? Can you continue to leave food for an animal which has been incapacitated for some time, until it is fully able to adapt to life in the wild again?

Birds

Short-term patients brought in with minor injuries should be released as soon as possible at the place where they were found, unless the site is clearly unsuitable. Birds which have been with you for a month or more will have considerable problems in readjusting to the wild and you *must* continue to offer food at the point of release (to which they will naturally return on a regular basis) until they no longer take it and are self-sufficient. On no account should you shrug off your responsibilities to the bird when you release it: your job is not yet complete and you must continue to support it as long as necessary.

If you have to take a bird to an area it does not know at all, keep it in its box or cage at the release point for at least an hour to let it get its bearings before it is freed. Release diurnal species early in the morning, preferably on a fine, warm day; release nocturnal species in the evening. For longer-term birds and hand-reared orphans, the best season for release (if there is any option) is spring or summer, when food supplies are abundant, but migrant species should obviously only be released in a season when they would be in Britain anyway, and preferably at the beginning of that season to give them ample time to prepare for migration.

With any passerine, think about habitat suitability and what the seasonal activities of the species would be at the time of release. With juvenile birds of all kinds, quality of habitat is much more important than returning to the place of origin. However, adult passerines of sedentary species should always be returned to the site of origin if feasible (they need a familiar environment), but for those of mobile species the quality of habitat is more important than familiarity.

With social (flocking) species, during the breeding season release into a known colony; in winter, release in a known feeding area; if you know of a roost, release just before dawn so that the bird can disperse with the crowd to contemporary feeding areas (it will undoubtedly be out of touch with local conditions).

Seabirds can be more difficult. Contact maritime organisations, local fishermen, local seabird clubs or rescue centres for advice on suitable season and site according to local conditions. Choose reasonable weather for the day of release.

The situation is more complicated with birds of prey and, as previously suggested, their rehabilitation should be handled by experts for both legal and practical reasons. The wildlife section of the Department of the Environment can give you the address of a suitable LRK. It is particularly important to continue to leave food for a released bird of prey at a recognised feeding station until it no longer makes use of it—and that could be for quite a long time.

Owls have similar rehabilitation requirements to diurnal raptors. To release captive-bred barn owlets, find a site which offers a suitable habitat in open farmland with plenty of hedgerows (barn owls are not a woodland species) and ample rodent life but no local use of rodenticides. Ideally you need about a hundred acres per owlet in good habitats. Persuade a friendly farmer (explain how useful the owls will be) to let a pair of owlets live in a sheltered, waterproof, undisturbed barn loft with a southerly to westerly aspect overlooking fields—ideally a square mile of open watermeadow with a few trees here and there and not a main road or electricity pylon in sight. Instal the birds in a "going-out" box in the loft at least 8 feet above ground level, with free access to the loft and out of it. The owlets, about six weeks old, will now need feeding: three whole day-old chicks each a night, and perhaps the farmer would undertake this small task if you supply the food. At eight or nine weeks old they will begin to try out their wings and need ample space within the loft for practice: check to see that they are not getting into trouble. By ten weeks old they will be flying well and further afield across the meadow but you must continue to feed them at the box because it can take up to two months for them to learn to hunt efficiently. You will probably need to go on feeding for a total of three months from the time the box was installed in the loft, just to make sure that they are given a really good start in life. Even then, continue to offer food for a few weeks in case they are not hunting too successfully.

An important factor in captive breed-and-release schemes is the introduction of new blood into a region in order to revitalise the local genetic pool of the species. If captive-bred birds are too closely related, the strain is weakened by inbreeding and it is therefore sensible to join a network of breed-and-releasers (such as BOBARS) so that, say, an owl from Dorset can be mated with one from Cambridge and the young released in Sussex to pair with local birds in the wild.

Mammals

In general, similar principles apply to release sites for mammals except that most of these animals, having their feet firmly on the ground, identify strongly with a familiar area. Make sure that that area is still suitable before you free the animal. The following species need special consideration.

Badgers   The badger is top of the list, and not only because it is first in alphabetical order. It is the rehabilitation factor which deters (or should deter) all but the experienced from rescuing and treating distressed badgers and your local badger group can tell you why.

Badgers live in extended families and they do *not* welcome strangers. The family is strongly territorial and an animal which loses its territory is at a severe disadvantage. A territory can be taken over during an absence of only two or three days. A released badger has a strong homing instinct and will make for its old sett but on the way there it will probably have to pass through other badger territories, at considerable disadvantage and risk, and then will no doubt find usurpers in its old home. However, individual badgers have been known to wander many, many miles in search of an acceptable territory, so let them do their own searching.

If an adult can be released straight into its original territory as quickly as possible, having been handled as little as possible in the meantime, it has a better chance of survival among its own tribe than elsewhere. However, an adult which has been a month or more in captivity will be a stranger in its own area and will be driven off by its own family.

A healthy "orphan" brought in by well-meaning rescuers should always be returned *immediately* to within 100 yards of the point where it was found. It then stands a chance of surviving and growing up within its tribe.

To select a suitable release site for hand-reared orphans, find a disused sett. If it is disused, then there is no resident in the territory but the fact that there is a sett at all indicates that the territory is (or was) capable of supporting a badger. However, find out *why* it is disused. Are there perhaps badger diggers in the area, or an MAFF TB-control programme? Only release the badger at the disused sett when you are satisfied that the territory remains suitable and safe. It may not stay there, preferring to try its luck elsewhere, but that must be its own decision.

Bats   Hand-reared juvenile bats should not be released, nor should you release adults after as much as twenty days in captivity: they will be out of touch with changes in local food sources and will waste so much energy searching unsuccessfully that they will almost certainly die, or alternatively they will have become so used to captivity that the colony will reject them.

If adults can be released in a much shorter time, take them to the place where they were originally found and free them at dusk, when insect densities are highest, or a little before sunset in cooler months so that it is less cold.

Permanently disabled bats usually adapt well to lifelong captivity and handling, which means that they can play an important role in educating the public. Make quite sure you have had the full agreement of the NCC at all stages of bat rescue.

Deer   Deer should only be released in an area where you are fairly sure they will not be the victims of the hunt, poachers, traffic, irate foresters or farmers, and also where they can find their own kind. They should never be transported to a site after recovery: it will probably kill them to be handled and confined for the journey. Release from the pen or paddock in which they have been recovering: simply open the gate and let them find their own way to freedom. You can leave hay and other food if you wish but they are unlikely to come back once they are free.

Do not release hand-reared deer into the wild. They will raid gardens even more rapaciously than wild deer and, being fearless of people, they will either injure someone or walk straight into a gun.

Foxes   Reared cubs can be allowed to wander off of their own accord from their shed or pen if the area is suitable but always with the option to return for food and shelter at will. The cub will probably explore an area within about 500 yards of the pen during the summer, improving its hunting skills all the while, and clearly the release point should therefore be in an area well away from gamekeepers, poultry keepers and hunts. Sadly, a lot of people consider that foxes are vermin to be destroyed on sight, and these beautiful animals have no protection from the law.

From August onwards the cub will explore further afield to find its own home ground. This might be within a mile of the release point, or perhaps as much as twenty-five miles away, though some cubs remain faithful to their original area. There will be risks for the young animal among its own kind. Foxes are strictly territorial and a newcomer will be chased from one area to another with little chance of settling and getting to know a territory, but that is a chance it would have to take even if raised in the wild by its own mother.

Adult foxes should be returned to their own territory as quickly as possible: nature really does abhor a vaccuum and another fox will soon move in.

Hedgehogs   Release hedgehogs only into areas where there are other hedgehogs, as this a good indication that the habitat is suitable for the species. Gardens are often good places, but there need to be several preferably with plenty of friendly owners who are fairly untidy gardeners and prepared to let hibernators rest in peace. Nor should there be any busy roads, pollution or badgers (one of the few animals capable of tackling a hedgehog). Home territory is best of all, with its familiar feeding places, hiding places and hazards, unless of course the cause of the hedgehog's original distress is still lurking. Leave a comfortable nesting box at the release point for a while until the animal has found its own quarters. If the release is shortly before hibernation time, make sure the hedgehog is plump enough for the winter and has access to lots of dead leaves so that it can build its nest in a compost heap or somewhere equally snug.

Mink   Do not release mink in the wild. They are not native to Britain, though many have escaped and thrive at the expense of the indigenous wildlife. Heed the example of the introduced grey squirrel.

Otters   The needs of wild otters are special and complex: for help and advice talk to the Otter Trust in Suffolk or the Vincent Wildlife Trust in Scotland. Captive-bred or hand-reared young otters must be able to fend for themselves before they are released, of course, but the main problem is finding the right habitat—unpolluted water, plenty of fish (and not guarded by water bailiffs!), lots of natural cover and the minimum of disturbance. As with other species, be suspicious if there are no otters in an apparently ideal area: there must be a good reason for their absence. Always consult private owners of suitable habitats and get their full and positive support before even considering releasing an otter.

Seals   This again is one for the experts. Let them choose the release point, the right weather and season, and hire the boats and the manpower to help transport these heavy mammals. There are several seal centres in Chapter 11, or you can contact the RSPCA or SSPCA.

CHAPTER TEN

THE LAW

There is a great deal of legislation concerning all kinds of animals, domesticated and wild, and clearly there is only enough space here to give selective and very broad generalisations about the ways in which these Acts might affect you or the animals you handle. The most directly relevant for many people is the Wildlife and Countryside Act 1981 which is a complex piece of legislation still not entirely understood even by the Department of the Environment (DOE), whom I have asked to give guidance in the context of this book in consultation with the Nature Conservancy Council (NCC). These two bodies are responsible for much of the administration and monitoring of the Act.

Wildlife and Countryside Act 1981 (WCA)

In so far as animal rescue is concerned, many people are alarmed that the very act of taking a distressed animal into their care might be a contravention of the WCA, especially in the case of Schedule 1 and Schedule 4 birds or Schedule 5 animals. (See Appendix 4 for a breakdown of species protected under the schedules of the WCA.) The Act was designed in the interests of conservation and it is an offence to kill, injure *or take* any wild bird, or to disturb a nesting Schedule 1 bird or its dependent young, except by special licence in certain circumstances. It is an offence to kill, injure or take any Schedule 5 animal *intentionally,* except by licence, or to possess or control such an animal, live or dead. However, you are absolved from such guilt if you have taken a disabled animal in order to tend and *release* it, or killed it because it was so seriously disabled that it had no reasonable chance of recovery. But if the casualty is a Schedule 4 bird, it must be registered with the DOE, which means it must be ringed by an LRK or under the care of a licensed veterinary surgeon.

Typical questions that you might have concerning the working of the Act are answered below by the DOE's Wildlife Division in Bristol in consultation with the NCC:

1. *What is the situation if I take in a distressed wild creature in order to care for it?*

It is not illegal for an individual to take any disabled wild bird, or any disabled animal normally protected under Section 9 of the Wildlife and Countryside Act 1981, provided that the bird or animal has not been disabled by that individual and as long as the disabled bird or animal is released back to the wild again when rehabilitated.

2.   *What if it should prove necessary to destroy the animal by approved humane methods?*

It is not illegal to kill a wild bird, or an animal protected under Section 9 of the 1981 Act as long as it can be shown that the bird or animal had been so seriously disabled other than by the individual's unlawful act and there was no reasonable chance of its recovering.

3.   *What if an individual accepts wildlife casualties from other people who cannot cope with a situation themselves?*

This is a little more complicated. It is likely that someone taking in an accident casualty which has been discovered by a third party would be covered as in (1) above. What is less clear is that person's position if the casualty has been disabled by an unlawful act by the third party. It would be sensible to conclude that they would have no way of knowing either way, but this is purely an opinion and it may be for a court to decide.

4.   *Is there any form of licensing or registration, apart from the LRK licence regarding Schedule 4 birds, which is required of any person or organisation seeking to take in and treat wildlife casualties of whatever species, and in particular is there any way in which a member of the public can be satisfied that such a person or organisation is in fact both permitted and competent to undertake such treatment?*

It would seem from the 1981 Act that there is no licensing requirement as long as an animal is taken for rehabilitation pending its release back to the wild. It would, therefore, be difficult for a member of the public to assess the capability of animal treatment centres. Perhaps the RSPCA could advise.

5.   *At what stage is a casualty decreed to be fit for release?*

This would possibly be a matter for the courts to decide.

6.   *Is there a register of competent rehabilitation centres?*

No such register exists.

7.   *How do I know if a bird of prey is registered with the DOE?*

The bird's leg will be fitted with a DOE close ring or plastic band carrying a unique number. All birds of prey, excluding owls, must be so registered.

8.   *What is an LRK?*

A Licensed Rehabilitation Keeper. The purpose of an LRK licence is to allow certain people who have the facilities, experience and expertise to tend birds and *successfully release them back to the wild,*to keep certain species of disabled registrable birds for up to six weeks without the need to register and ring them. If the bird is unable to be released after six weeks, then it must be registered with the DOE and, if necessary, ringed. It should be stressed that this is *not* a licence to treat birds (such a licence is unnecessary), nor does it permit the taking of any wild bird from the wild, nor is it evidence that the bird was legally taken from the wild or is held legally. Neither the licence itself, nor subsequent registration of the bird, conveys any right of ownership of the bird being kept. If a bird taken in because of some other disability subsequently becomes imprinted on humans and cannot be released to the wild, the DOE would normally consider that the LRK has failed in the duty to help the bird recover. LRKs are expected to take steps to ensure imprinting does not occur. Veterinary surgeons and practitioners are covered by the DOE's general licence to keep unregistered or registered Schedule 4 birds for a period of up to six weeks (provided such birds are undergoing treatment or care) without having to register and ring them. For advice on fitting a DOE ring, and on all aspects of being an LRK, contact the DOE's Wildlife Division in Bristol (address in Appendix 5).

A couple of other points from the WCA need to be noted. For example, you are not supposed to release into the wild non-native species such as Canada geese, coypu, mink or grey squirrels. If a wildlife rescue centre kept all its squirrel casualties, it would be overrun within the month!

There is also the question of cages for birds. The Act states that a cage or other means of confinement for the bird must give it enough space to stretch its wings freely. This requirement is not laid upon veterinary surgeons who are examining or treating a bird but it *does* apply to lay people caring for a bird: any container used by a lay person to confine a wild bird must allow it to stretch its wings, even if it is a hospital cage. If, therefore, you deem it necessary in the bird's best interests that its ability to spread its wings should be limited, you must put the bird under the care of a vet.

Following from that, you should know that under the terms of the Veterinary Surgeons Act 1966 your status as a non-veterinarian treating animal casualties is in some doubt. You should always entrust a domestic animal to the care of a qualified vet for diagnosis and treatment, but the situation with sick or injured free-living wild animals is less clear, though you can certainly give emergency first aid on the spot. However, in order to give any further treatment to a wild animal you have to become its "owner" which means that you exercise some form of control over it. Only then are you able to give it veterinary treatment or to ask a vet to treat it, and if you ask a non-veterinarian at a wildlife rescue centre to treat it, then you must hand over the "ownership" to the centre. What it really boils down to is that if any kind of animal, wild or domesticated, is in trouble, anybody can give it emergency first aid but thereafter it is both practically and morally advisable to consult a qualified veterinary practice for proper diagnosis and treatment, or advice on treatment. That is what vets are trained to do, and you are not. It is also likely that drugs will be needed, and usually these can only be obtained on prescription by a vet, and only for animals which are under the vet's care—and that means a real rather than nominal responsibility for the animal.

Road Traffic Accidents

Livestock and dogs   If a vehicle on a public road is involved in an accident which causes death or injury to cattle, horses, asses, mules, sheep, goats, pigs or dogs, the driver is obliged to stop and help, and also to try and find the animal's owner and give that person the name and address of the driver and of the vehicle's owner, along with the vehicle's registration number. The owner then becomes responsible for dealing with the animal. If the owner cannot be located, the police must be notified immediately so that they can take the responsibility for bringing veterinary assistance to an injured animal, which might include its humane destruction if necessary.

Cats and other domesticated animals   No legal obligation to report an accident.

Wild species   No legal obligation to report the death or injury of a wild animal unless it is a protected species (see WCA), in which case the police *must* be notified.

Abandonment of Animals Act 1960

This Act, although designed to protect pets from being deserted, also applies to wildlife rescuers in that it covers rehabilitated wild animals or those bred in captivity for the purpose of boosting the wild population. The effect of the Act is that you must make a very careful assessment of the animal's ability to survive in the wild before it is released, which means checking its physical condition and also the environment into which it will be released.

Cruelty

There are many laws seeking to protect the welfare of all kinds of animals. Any domestic or *captive* animal, for example, is covered by the Protection of Animals Acts 1911-1964, be it mammal, bird, fish or reptile, but the concept of captivity does not include, say, an animal restrained by a hunter while it is killed, though many wild animals are protected from being so killed under the WCA, and some also receive protection under special legislation, particularly badgers.

The 1973 Badgers Act, in combination with the WCA, makes cruelty to badgers illegal including ill-treatment in general (and, specifically, the use of weapons other than specified calibre rifles), the use of badger tongs, and badger-digging. While it is an offence to dig *for* a badger, it is not necessarily illegal to dig in, stop or otherwise disturb a sett—which seems illogical.

Dangerous Species

A dangerous species, as defined by the Animals Act 1971, is one which is not commonly domesticated in the British Isles and the adults of which normally have such characteristics that they are likely to cause severe damage unless restrained. This could include, say, a stag and certainly any exotic carnivores such as the big cats, even if they are claimed to be "tame" (tameness and domestication are not the same). The keeper of a dangerous animal is wholly liable for any harm caused by it, even if the individual animal has had no previous record or obvious ability to cause damage. It would be better if this legislation also included hand-reared male deer, since they are known to be dangerous because of their lack of fear of humans.

Diseases

Certain contagious diseases are classified as notifiable, that is, if an animal is diagnosed as suffering from or carrying such a disease, or even suspected of being a case, it must be reported to the police or the local veterinary division of the Ministry of Agriculture, Fisheries and Food (MAFF). Under the Animal Health Act 1981, these rules normally apply to farm livestock but they also concern other species affected by similar diseases (for example, foot-and-mouth affects deer as well as cattle) and MAFF are empowered to destroy wildlife to prevent the spread of certain diseases where necessary—the controversial killing of badgers accused of transmitting tuberculosis to cattle is one such example. Although most of the orders relating to notifiable diseases are limited to domesticated species, some have much wider coverage—anthrax, rabies, cattle plague, foot-and-mouth disease, zoonotic diseases (those which can be transmitted to humans), fish diseases, and bird diseases like psittacosis, ornithosis, Newcastle disease, fowl plague and pigeon paramyxovirus. Salmonella and brucella organisms in many species are reportable under the Zoonoses Order 1975 in animals produced for human consumption, and MAFF might also investigate outbreaks in any other species as well.

Licences

Wherever there is a law, there seem to be exceptions to it if you can get an appropriate licence. For example, the general rule that you may not kill or take certain birds can be waived if you obtain a licence from an appropriate government department. This might be for the purpose of ringing or marking, conservation, protecting a collection of wild animals, practising falconry or aviculture, selling certain protected wild species and so on. In most cases the licences are obtainable from DOE, NCC or MAFF.

Transport

The legislation on transport of animals refers largely to domesticated species, especially farm livestock. However, an article in the Transit of Animals (General) Order 1973, which includes any species you can think of (mammals, fish, reptiles, crustaceans and other cold-blooded animals, excluding poultry and farm animals covered by other orders) by any means of transport on land, sea or air, makes it an offence to transport an animal which is unfit or likely to give birth during the journey. While clearly it is nonsense not to be able to transport a sick animal to a veterinary surgery for treatment, the article has been used by a public transport concern to refuse to convey sick animals to a wildlife hospital.

CHAPTER ELEVEN

THE RESCUERS

All sciences can easily be learned by any man; but understanding is a gift of God, and it comes only to those who keep their hearts open.

William J. Long, *How Animals Talk,* 1919

In every corner of this land there are people who devote their lives to the care of distressed animals. Some of the rescuers are within major charities, with centres all over the country and perhaps abroad as well, supported entirely by gifts from members of the public. The great majority, however, are back-gardeners who once tried to nurse a fledgling or care for a partly squashed hedgehog found by the roadside, and who then became the neighbourhood focus for all kinds of injured wildlife, or people who rescued a half-drowned litter of kittens, or saw a lost and half-starved dog whose eyes met theirs and they took it home to restore some of its faith in humanity.

From such individual incidents did the big charities spring but most will remain personal sanctuaries where caring people battle to keep many lives going and to improve the quality of those lives. Without exception these casualty tenders are overwhelmed by the numbers of creatures brought to them for help and it would ease their burdens if more people were willing and competent to handle at least the cases which require patience and application rather than skill and experience.

There are countless ways in which those who are unable to commit themselves to the full-time care of distressed animals could help those who do take them in. Money is always needed—for food, veterinary fees and medical supplies above all—or appropriate gifts in kind on a regular basis. As important is practical help, like acting as chauffeur to bring in casualties from those who have no means of transport, or becoming involved with rehoming, rehabilitation and release schemes, or just helping with cleaning out and routine feeding, or becoming trained in more skilful work including rescue techniques and first aid so that, once in a while, the centre's owners can take a break. If you *can* offer practical help of any kind, however limited or mundane, remember that the owners are working for love and with total commitment: be prepared to offer regular and absolutely reliable support when it is needed, so that they and the animals can rely on you.

In the following pages there are the names, addresses and details of a wide range of people, groups and organisations involved in all aspects of animal rescue. They represent only a fraction of the compassionate army: there are probably thousands more like them, quietly getting on with the life's work they have set themselves, some of them living in the wilder parts of the country, some on farms or in rural villages, many in the suburbs of towns and some in little oases in the heart of the city. They are in most cases willing to take in distressed animals without question or to give advice if you want to care for an animal yourself. It is always worth consulting the major charities, who will usually know something about the more reliable and experienced individuals as well as having their own rescue centres in many cases.

MAJOR NATIONAL AND INTERNATIONAL ORGANISATIONS

ANIMAL AID, 7 Castle Street, Tonbridge, Kent TN9 1BH
Telephone: 0732 364546
A campaigning and educational organisation formed in 1977 to oppose the abuse of animals, particularly in vivisection laboratories and factory farms. Active but non-violent campaigning. No facilities for treating or sheltering animals but can give advice on relevant organisations to approach.
Journal: *Outrage.*

ANIMAL CONCERN (SCOTLAND), 121 West Regent Street, Glasgow G2 2SD   Telephone: 041 221 2300
Animal rights group campaigning against animal exploitation in general; no facilities for care and treatment of distressed animals.
Journal: *News.*

ANIMAL WELFARE TRUST, Tyler's Way, Watford By-pass, Watford, Herts WD2 8HQ   Telephone: 01 950 8215/0177
Set up in 1971 to care for animals which are neglected, abused or unwanted. Principal work is to find homes for dogs, cats and other pets—rescues and rehomes thousands each year and never puts down a healthy animal. Has own rescue centre near Watford, with arrangements for boarding and rehoming in Birmingham, Ipswich and Bristol. Works closely with other welfare organisations and breed rescue groups. Mostly domesticated species including small livestock and poultry; mostly for sanctuary and rehoming, but often takes in casualties, including a few wild species. Formed Pet Concern scheme in 1979 to give financial assistance towards boarding fees for pets

of senior citizens and disabled; also emergency pet care scheme ensuring pets are cared for in short-term emergencies. Adopt-an-animal sponsorship scheme and other fund-raising activities. Registered charity.
Journal: *Bulletin.*

THE DOGS' HOME, BATTERSEA, 4 Battersea Park Road, London SW8 4AA   Telephone: 01 622 3626
World-famous dogs' home—takes in about 23,000 dogs a year of which about three-quarters are either reclaimed by their owners or found new homes; the rest are destroyed. Spays and neuters about 2,000 animals each year. Contractually obliged to offer shelter to stray dogs taken into police custody (sometimes up to 70 new dogs a day). Registered charity. Quarterly newsletter.

THE BLUE CROSS, The Animals' Hospital, Hugh Street, Victoria, London SW1V 1QQ   Telephone: 01 834 4224/5556
Practical animal welfare group with own veterinary facilities, mainly for dogs, cats, horses, and finds new homes for large numbers of pet animals. Cares for strays that are sick and injured and also provides free treatment for animals whose owners cannot afford private veterinary fees. Main clinical centre in Victoria; major new Field Centre at Home Close Farm, Shilton Road, Burford, Oxon, with kennels, stables, cattery, aviary etc.; also hospitals, catteries, kennels and other facilities in many parts of the country including Wandsworth, Hammersmith, Hertfordshire (mainly dogs), Chalfont St Peter (main welfare boarding facility for cats), Thirsk, Tiverton, Kimpton. Registered charity.
Journal: *Blue Cross Illustrated.*

BRITISH BIRD COUNCIL, 1577 Bristol Road South, Birmingham B45 9UA   Telephone: 021 4539284
Set up in 1971 by a group of breeders and exhibitors of captive British wild bird species to represent the interests of the British Bird Fancy. Took over the BBBA ringing system in 1971; adopted a unique continuous numbering system in 1976.

BRITISH HERPETOLOGICAL SOCIETY, c/o Zoological Society of London, Regent's Park, London NW1 4RY
Founded in 1947 with the broad aim of catering for all aspects of interest in reptiles and amphibians. Originally a small group of enthusiastic naturalists, now with national status and international connections. Forum for exchange of experiences in maintaining, breeding and observing various species in captivity or observation in the wild (including active conservation of native British species).

Journal: *Bulletin.*

BRITISH HORSE SOCIETY, British Equestrian Centre, Stoneleigh, Kenilworth, Warks CV8 2LR   Telephone: 0203 696697
Works for the well-being of all horses and ponies. Has a National Equine Welfare Officer to monitor the interests of horses and ponies in riding and trekking establishments. Close liaison with the veterinary profession, RSPCA and SSPCA, the Donkey Sanctuary and other equine welfare societies. Nationwide network of welfare workers can be contacted locally if a horse is known to be in distress. Seeks to educate the horse-owning public— numerous publications, including codes of practice and guidelines on tethering, livery stables, horse-drawn caravans, motorway rescue service, euthanasia, auctions etc.

BRITISH OWL BREEDING AND RELEASE SCHEME (BOBARS), The Owl Centre, Muncaster Castle, Ravenglass, Cumbria CA18 1RQ   Telephone 06577 393
Tony Warburton's BOBARS project has been responsible for the release of more than 300 captive-bred barn owlets in the last fifteen years, aided by Peter Olney at London Zoo and a host of individual owl breeders, farmers and landowners. BOBARS can supply full details of nest-box design and siting, and of the stages of owlet release.

BRITISH TRUST FOR ORNITHOLOGY, Beech Grove, Station Road, Tring, Herts HP23 5NR   Telephone 044 2822 3461
More than fifty years old, the Trust aims to study the British wild bird population in all aspects, especially to see how birds are affected by human activities. Practical advice on conservation. Guidance and help for members' own studies, which often become co-ordinated national efforts (for example, work on sand martins, peregrines, herons, effects of DDT on raptors). Network of regional representatives and members throughout Britain. Close liaison with NCC, government departments, local authorities, conservation organisations. Substantial library and bird records at Tring: wide-ranging ringing system provides superb database. Financed by membership subscriptions and NCC contracts.
Journals: *BTO News, Bird Study, Ringing and Migration.*

BRITISH WATERFOWL ASSOCIATION, 6 Caldicott Close, Over, Winsford, Cheshire CW7 1LW   Telephone: 0606 594150
Association for those who keep, breed and conserve all types of waterfowl, including wildfowl and domestic ducks and geese. Dedicated to educating the public about waterfowl in general and the need for conservation; also raising standards of keeping and breeding ducks, geese and swans in captivity.

Access to a panel of experts. Annual show and sale in conjunction with Rare Breeds Survival Trust at Stoneleigh. Registered charity. Annual waterfowl yearbook and buyers' guide.
Journal: *Waterfowl.*

BRITISH WILDLIFE REHABILITATION COUNCIL,

c/o Wildlife Hospitals Trust, 1 Pemberton Close, Aylesbury, Bucks HP21 7NY   Telephone (c/o RSPCA): 0403 64181
Organisation set up in 1987 to encourage contact and exchange of information between all those involved in rehabilitation of sick, orphaned and injured native vertebrate animals and to promote the humane care of those species by the dissemination of information. Central point of contact for rehabilitators, veterinary surgeons, relevant welfare organisations and others involved in wildlife rescue work with the emphasis on rehabilitation. It is still in formative stages at the time of writing but has big ideas and considerable support.

CATS PROTECTION LEAGUE, 17 Kings Road, Horsham, West

Sussex RH13 5PP   Telephone: 0403 65566
Cat welfare charity started in 1927 with the aim of educating cat owners to their responsibilities, including the advisability of neutering and spaying. Became national in the late 1970s and now has 185 groups and branches nationwide, manned by voluntary workers. Eight large rescue centres, mainly concerned with rehoming cats. Sponsorship scheme for unhomeable animals, though the main work is providing temporary transit accommodation for needy and unwanted cats whilst new homes are found. Publishes good range of freely available literature in the cause of better and more responsible cat care. Registered charity entirely dependent upon subscriptions, donations and legacies.
Journal: *The Cat.*

COMPASSION IN WORLD FARMING, 20 Lavant Street,

Petersfield, Hants GU32 3EW   Telephone: 0730 64208
Public trust founded in 1967 concerned with the agricultural and food aspects of the total environment: seeks to introduce non-violence into human relationships with farm animals, wildlife and the plant kingdom. Particularly concerned with unwitting abuse of farm animals by environmental and behavioural deprivation in intensive systems, the export of live food animals, and careless practices during "humane" slaughter; also seeks more humane treatment of "pest" species (for example, contraceptive bait techniques instead of poisons). No facilities for practical animal rescue.
Journal: *Agscene.*

THE DONKEY SANCTUARY, Sidmouth, Devon EX10 0NU
Telephone: 03955 6391/78222
Very famous donkey sanctuary, started at Ottery St Mary in 1969 by Mrs Elisabeth Svendsen; became a registered charity in 1973. Hospital and intensive care unit opened 1982. Now has almost a thousand acres, catering for more than 3,000 rescued donkeys on a permanent basis. Geriatric units for ageing donkeys where they can spend the rest of their days. Educational literature and lectures. Six full-time inspectors and 52 trained voluntary staff cover the whole country to monitor markets and follow up reports of cruelty, also liaison with local councils where donkeys are being used for profit. Relies entirely on public donations. Two other registered charities from same address: **The International Donkey Protection Trust,** which works throughout the world, and **The Slade Centre,** which helps handicapped children to enjoy and ride donkeys. Visitors (free admission) 9 a.m. to dusk daily.

GLENDA SPOONER TRUST: HORSES AND PONIES IN NEED, Emmetts Hill, Whichford, Warks CV36 5PG
Telephone: 0608 84683
Founded in 1987 to try and prevent ill-treatment of all horses and ponies and to alleviate suffering. Works to increase public awareness of cruelty and exploitation, and to advise, inform and educate in the interests of good equine management. Acts in co-operation with local authorities and welfare organisations to investigate and take positive action in cases of equine distress of any kind. Prepared to undertake prosecutions where necessary. Will buy seriously distressed animal if it has a good chance of rehabilitation or requires humane destruction. Willing to advise and help with any problems, and works with other welfare organisations with similar objectives. Registered charity.

GREENPEACE, 30-31 Islington Green, London N1 8BR
Telephone: 01 354 5100
International environmental pressure group, independent of all political parties. Campaigns too numerous to mention, but of particular relevance are its activities to protect whales, seals, dolphins and porpoises. Helps RSPCA with the rescue of virus-stricken seals. Uses peaceful direct action to invoke the power of public opinion as a major weapon in changing laws to protect wildlife and stop pollution of the natural world.
Quarterly journal: *Greenpeace News.*

GUERNSEY SOCIETY FOR THE PREVENTION OF CRUELTY TO ANIMALS, The Animal Shelter, Les Fiers Moutons, St Andrew's, Guernsey, CI   Telephone: 0481 57261
Founded in 1873. Aims to rescue all animals and birds in distress or danger, return to own homes where possible if lost, find new homes for strays or

those needing rehousing, take care of wounded or ailing creatures, rehabilitate wild creatures when fit. Help and advice on care of pets and working animals. Trains a team of voluntary wardens; very useful warden's manual.

HAWK TRUST, c/o Birds of Prey Section, Zoological Society of London, Regent's Park, London NE1 4RY   Telephone: 01 722 3333
Valuable source of information on birds of prey. Recently opened a National Centre for Owl Conservation at Blickling Estate, Aylsham, Norfolk, to increase public awareness of the barn owl's fight for survival. Offers information on nest-box siting and construction.

HEARING DOGS FOR THE DEAF, (Training Centre) London Road, Lewknor, Oxon OX9 5RY   Telephone: 0844 53898
Charity assisting people who have suffered loss of hearing by training dogs to respond to everyday sounds. Gives unwanted mongrels the chance of a very good home and an important role as their new owners' "ears". Journal: *Favour.*

HORSES AND PONIES PROTECTION ASSOCIATION, Greenbank Farm, Greenbank Drive, Fence, Burnley, Lancs BB12 9QP   Telephone: 0282 65909
Specialises in rescuing cruelly treated and neglected horses, ponies and donkeys. Three full-time field officers (ex-mounted police) and four part-time officers to investigate complaints. Three farms where animals are cared for during recovery. Fully recovered animals can be loaned (never sold) to carefully assessed homes under legal agreement. HAPPA investigates and frequently prosecutes in cases of cruelty, offers advice service for horse and pony owners, campaigns for better legislation to prevent suffering and operates a lost-and-found register. Registered charity.

HUMANE EDUCATION CENTRE, Bounds Green Road, London N22 4EU   Telephone: 01 889 1595
The first centre of its kind in the United Kingdom set up with the specific aim of promoting among all ages humane treatment of animals.

HUMANE SLAUGHTER ASSOCIATION, 34 Blanche Lane, South Mimms, Potters Bar, Herts EN6 3PA   Telephone: 0707 59040
Independent, objective and rational animal welfare charity seeking to improve transportation, marketing and slaughter conditions for all farm animals.

INTERNATIONAL LEAGUE FOR THE PROTECTION OF HORSES, 67a Camden High Street, London NW1 7JL
Telephone: 01 388 1449/8333
Instrumental in introducing legislation in respect of horses being exported

for slaughter. Has purchased thousands of distressed horses, and brought them back to health wherever possible so that they can be found good homes. Widely known rest and rehabilitation centres in Surrey, Norfolk and Dublin, as well as a veterinary clinic in the Moroccan province of Agadir and branches in many overseas countries. Field officers cover the whole of Britain to investigate complaints about ill-treatment of horses and donkeys. Will respond speedily to calls for help or advice, but members of the public should not take casualties to any of the centres without a preliminary telephone call. Registered charity.

INTERNATIONAL WILDLIFE REHABILITATION COUNCIL, PO Box 3007, Walnut Creek, California, USA 94598

There are probably about 3,000 individually licensed wildlife rehabilitators in America today and IWRC is an association of professional wildlife carers which holds training classes, publishes many special papers on wildlife rehabilitation and a quarterly journal. Several of its member centres produce literature to educate the public as they get frequent calls for help and advice on various species. The association also has members in Canada, South America, Europe, Australia and Mexico and would welcome articles on British species and rehabilitators in Britain.

LEAGUE AGAINST CRUEL SPORTS, Sparling House, 83-87 Union Street, London SE1 1SG   Telephone: 01 407 0979

The League's role is to campaign for the legal protection of wildlife from the infliction of unnecessary suffering. Seeks to use educational and public relations methods to further its aims, approaches landowners direct to ask them to prohibit hunting and unnecessary shooting on their land, offers a free legal service to those whose land has been invaded by hounds and mounted followers, and buys land in order to protect wildlife (largely in Devon and Somerset, where red deer are hunted with dogs). Gives advice and sometimes practical assistance for "moving on" unwelcome urban foxes, and offers sensible advice on how to handle situations in which you believe unnecessary suffering is being inflicted on wild animals, making sure that your own actions remains well within the law.

NATIONAL ANIMAL RESCUE ASSOCIATION, 8 Waterpump Court, Thorplands, Northampton NN3 1XU Telephone: 0604 494602

An emergency and rescue service operating in the field—NARA takes help to sick, trapped and injured animals wherever they are found. Manned by volunteers on call twenty-four hours a day every day of the year. Maintains emergency ambulances and rescue boats; has an army of trained volunteers all over Britain prepared to respond to any call for help in any situation—

including a fully trained parachute and helicopter unit to respond to any animal disaster zone, irrespective of the difficulties involved.

NARA has produced an invaluable animal first-aid manual written by Rorke S. Garfield. The association relies entirely on local community support and volunteers. Registered charity.

NATIONAL CANINE DEFENCE LEAGUE, 1 & 2 Pratt Mews, London NW1 0AD   Telephone: 01 388 0137
NCDL has been fighting on the side of dogs for a century, taking an active interest in any legislation which affects dogs, and giving awards to life-saving or otherwise heroic dogs. Maintains rescue centres all over Britain, finds new homes for unwanted dogs and tries to ensure that all dogs are properly identified so that owners can be relocated if the dogs stray. Runs sponsorship schemes. Registered charity.

NATIONAL EQUINE (AND SMALLER ANIMALS) DEFENCE LEAGUE, The Animals' Refuge and Hospital, Oak Tree Farm, Wetheral Shields, Carlisle CA4 8JA   Telephone: 0228 60082
Founded in 1909, the League is involved in many aspects of animal welfare work and is especially active in publishing educational material. As well as homes of rest for horses, the Oak Tree Farm complex houses many smaller animal species, domesticated and wild. Wild species are accepted for treatment with the intention of rehabilitation, though disabled birds are retained in aviaries designed to give as natural an environment as possible. All sorts of animals receive veterinary treatment in the Oak Tree Farm hospital unit, which includes an intensive care unit and an isolation area for those with infectious diseases. Registered charity.

NATURE CONSERVANCY COUNCIL, Northminster House, Northminster, Peterborough, Cambs PE1 1UA *or* Hope Terrace, Edinburgh EH9 2AS   Telephone: 0733 40345 (Peterborough)
Government-funded national organisation which promotes nature conservation and actively protects wildlife habitats, managing nature reserves all over the country. Local offices can give advice on wildlife matters of all kinds, especially environmental. many useful publications

PEOPLE'S DISPENSARY FOR SICK ANIMALS,
PDSA House, South Street, Dorking, Surrey RH4 2LB
Telephone: 0306 888291
Founded in 1917 in the slums of London by Maria Dickin with the intention of providing free treatment for animals whose owners could least afford it. Since then, the organisation has been specifically charged by Parliament (in

the PDSA Act) to spend its resources only on those who genuinely need help. However, they have also introduced a pet insurance scheme for those dog and cat owners who have no access to existing PDSA services. The PDSA animal treatment centres in many towns now treat more than a million animals a year, and more are treated by the Auxiliary Service launched in 1980. Between them, these services and clinics cover about a hundred towns. Registered charity.

PETWATCH, PO Box 16, Brighouse, West Yorkshire HD6 1DS
Telephone: 0484 722411
Unique charity set up in 1983 to deal specifically with the growing problem of stolen family pets. Basic aim is to protect pet animals from ill-usage, cruelty and suffering and to encourage the development and administration of the law in respect of the theft of pets. Works closely with all the major and local animal welfare groups, the police and various international organisations, and gives advice and practical help to owners whose pets are missing—where to look, where to advertise, who needs to be informed or contacted. Maintains local missing pets registers in many areas. Registered charity.

ROYAL PIGEON RACING ASSOCIATION, The Reddings,
Cheltenham, Glos GL51 6RN   Telephone: 0452 713529
If you find a pigeon with a ring on its leg, and it fails to fly off in due course, its owner can be traced if you report the ring number to the Royal Pigeon Racing Assocation. If the number includes "Wales", the bird is registered with the Welsh Homing Union; NEHU is the North of England Homing Union; SHU and IHU the Scottish and Irish unions respectively. Foreign birds can also be traced on what the RPRA calls its "Chinese" list. Will advise you on the proper procedures for returning the bird to its owner and looking after it in the meantime.

**ROYAL SOCIETY FOR THE PREVENTION OF CRUELTY
TO ANIMALS,** Causeway, Horsham, West Sussex RH12 1HG
Telephone: 0403 64181
Established in 1824. The only organisation which covers every aspect of animal welfare, whether the animals are wild, domesticated, captive, farm livestock or in the laboratory. The scope of its work hardly needs description: 230 inspectors, 150 animal homes, centres and clinics throughout England and Wales. The Horsham address is its headquarters, and is also the home of the Wildlife Department. The organisation is huge, and for that reason it has a substantial database of information about the care and rehabilitation of animals of all kinds—a very useful source of experienced advice. Addresses and telephone numbers of trained inspectors can be found in your local telephone directory: they will treat all complaints about cruelty in strict

confidence and will take every possible step to prevent cruelty, whether it has been deliberately inflicted or has occurred simply as a result of ignorance or neglect.

Wildlife casualties of all kinds can be treated (but not given permanent homes) by the **Wildlife Field Unit** at Little Creech Farm, West Hatch, near the Somerset town of Taunton. The unit deals with more than 2,000 animals a year of at least 80 different species and has a specialist cleaning system for oiled birds. It is well equipped to deal with most situations or to give advice on matters relating to animal welfare, but resources and the number of personnel are limited so do not bother them with simple queries during peak seasons. There is also a **Wildlife Sanctuary and Field Study Centre** at Mallydams Wood, Peter James Lane, Fairlight, near Hastings in East Sussex.

Seals are dealt with by a new special seal assessment and emergency rescue unit set up to try and deal with the 1988 viral epidemic. The unit is at Northcote, Docking, Fakenham, Norfolk (04858 209).

The **SCOTTISH SPCA** deals with a different range of wild birds and animals and has a special oiled-bird cleaning centre at Inverkeithing. Its headquarters are to be found at 19 Melville Street, Edinburgh EH3 7PL.

ROYAL SOCIETY FOR THE PROTECTION OF BIRDS,
The Lodge, Sandy, Bedfordshire SG19 2DL   Telephone: 0767 80551
The largest voluntary wildlife conservation organisation in Europe, with a membership of over half a million people. RSPB owns or leases more than a hundred reserves and it is devoted to the conservation and protection of wild birds—*in the wild.* That means it is also concerned with bird habitats, but it is *not* involved in welfare, bird hospitals, the killing of gamebirds, caged birds or falconry. Welfare issues are handled by the RSPCA and other specialist welfare organisations: the RSPB does not have trained veterinary staff, nor does it have the time, funds or inclination to monitor wild-bird hospitals or investigate factory farming of poultry.

SWAN RESCUE SERVICE EUROPE, Shotesham St Mary,
Norwich, Norfolk NR15 1XX   Telephone: 050842 248/8357
Len Baker is one of four full-time volunteers who make sure that the Swan Rescue telephone is answered at quite literally any time of the day or night, although there has recently been some doubt about the continuation of this service. There are also six part-time volunteers and they are prepared to go anywhere in the British Isles or in Europe for the sake of injured or sick swans, relying entirely on donations to keep the service running. They would welcome local "look-outs" to cover various areas of the country. They have a swan sanctuary and hospital in Norfolk.

UNIVERSITIES FEDERATION FOR ANIMAL WELFARE,

8 Hamilton Close, South Mimms, Potters Bar, Herts EN6 3QD
Telephone: 0707 58202
UFAW's aim is to promote the better treatment of all animals through
education by means of lectures, symposia, workshops and technical
publications. The federation has produced some classic welfare books,
especially those concerning the welfare of farm livestock and laboratory
animals, the humane control of wildlife, and humane killing of all species.

WHALE AND DOLPHIN CONSERVATION SOCIETY,

20 West Lea Road, Bath, Avon BA1 3RL   Telephone: 0225 334511
The only organisation in the United Kingdom devoted solely to the
conservation and welfare of all species of whales, dolphins and porpoises.
WDCS has campaigned on subjects such as the whaling industry, dolphins
in captivity and the killing of dolphins by the tuna–fishing industry. Contact
the society's volunteer executive director, Sean Whyte, for advice on stranded
whales and dolphins.
Journals: *Sonar* and *International Whale Bulletin.*

WILDFOWL TRUST, Slimbridge, Gloucester GL2 7BT

Telephone: 0453 890100
Founded by Sir Peter Scott in 1946 with the aim of protecting wildfowl
threatened with extinction, conserving wetland areas, and making it possible
for people to observe, enjoy and learn about birds and their environment.
Slimbridge is headquarters of the International Waterfowl Research Bureau.
Other reserves at Arundel, Caerlaverock, Martin Mere, Peakirk, Washington,
Welney. If you need advice on wildfowl, become a member. Non-profit
making, and dependent on members' subscriptions, donations and sponsorship.
Journal: *Wildfowl World.*

WILDLIFE HOSPITALS TRUST (ST TIGGYWINKLES),

1 Pemberton Close, Aylesbury, Bucks HP21 7NY
Telephone: 0296 29860
Les and Sue Stocker specialise in trying to save wildlife—all species, including
of course hedgehogs about which the Stockers must know more than
anybody. Rehabilitation is their aim, releasing patients back into the wild as
soon as possible. Hospital facilities in Aylesbury are good, and they are now
aiming to establish Europe's first wildlife teaching hospital. In the meantime,
they will accept (or arrange to collect) hedgehog casualties from all over the
country. But they will accept *all* species of British wildlife, including the
pigeons, sparrows and rodents other wildlife rescuers might not want to
accommodate.

WOOD GREEN ANIMAL SHELTERS, Highway Cottage, Chishill
Road, Heydon, Royston, Herts SG8 8PN
Telephone: 0763 838329
Established in 1924 and now with three centres: at 601 Lordship Lane, Wood
Green, London N22; at Heydon; and at the Margaret Young Home for
Animals, King's Bush Farm, London Road, Godmanchester, Huntingdon,
which they believe is the most up to date in Europe. They take in anything
from dogs and cats to horses, goats and sheep—cruelty cases, abandoned or
neglected animals, victims of RTAs and other accidents, and animals which
can no longer be accommodated by their owners. Will train or retrain if
necessary for rehoming as many as possible. Variety of educational and
advisory services including riding for the disabled, animal visits for the elderly,
adopt–a–pet service etc. Registered charity.
Journal: *Animal Matters.*

WORLD SOCIETY FOR THE PROTECTION OF ANIMALS,
106 Jermyn Street, London SW1Y 6EE   Telephone: 01 839 3026
Claims to be "the world's widest ranging animal protection society". Over
350 member humane organisations in 60 countries as well as thousands of
individual members. All the major welfare groups in Britain are members
of this umbrella organisation. Actively involved in animal protection since
1959, WSPA works to protect all animal life—domestic pets, farm livestock,
wild animals, laboratory animals *et al.* Consultative status with the United
Nations; works through member societies and inter-governmental agencies
on an international scale. Organises animal rescues in major natural disasters;
campaigns against activities like whaling, bullfighting, kangaroo slaughter,
vivisection, fur trade, killing of any wild animal for commercial reasons,
inhumane conditions during transport and slaughter of food animals, exotic
pet trade. Registered charity.
Journal: *Animals International.*

RESCUE CENTRES

Full addresses and telephone numbers have in some cases been omitted, at
the request of the proprietor. The acronym "LRK" used throughout this
section means "Licensed Rehabilitation Keeper".

NOTE: For up-to-date information on bird hospitals, consult the current
edition of John Pemberton's *The Birdwatcher's Yearbook* (Buckingham Press).
There are several hundred centres for injured and sick birds in the United
Kingdom.

ABBOTSFORD SANCTUARY, 143 Church Road, Kessingland, Lowestoft, Suffolk
Proprietor: Mrs S. M. Wohlgemuth
All species of bird, especially seabirds (oiled or injured).

ADOPT-A-CAT, 62 Brighton Road, Shoreham by Sea, West Sussex BN4 6RG
Proprietor: Grace McHattie
Directory of cat sanctuaries and shelters all over the country. Sponsored by Go-Cat and Gourmet.

ANIMAL REHABILITATION CENTRE, East Midlands
Telephone: 0400 50246   Proprietor: Molly Burkett
The Burketts have been involved in wildlife rehabilitation since 1952; they can claim more than two thousand *successful* releases into the wild and their knowledge is extensive. They now act largely in an advisory capacity but will take any wild animal or bird on condition that it is to be released back to the wild if and when they think it is fit. They will only accept the animal if told exactly where it was found and whether there is someone willing and able to monitor its rehabilitation for several weeks after release. They emphasize the importance of keeping the creature wild—no other people are allowed contact with a Burkett patient.

BERKSHIRE WILDLIFE REHABILITATION UNIT, 8 Mill Lane, Padworth, Berkshire RG7 4JU
Telephone: 0734 712781   Proprietors: C. A. and R. J. Palmer
Formed in 1981, when the Palmers had already been caring for sick and injured raptors and other birds for nine years. Aims are to care for and rehabilitate injured birds and, where possible, to hack back to the wild; also to provide information to the general public about birds of prey in general. LRK. Members of BOBARS. Funded by personal resources, income from lectures, public donations and sponsorship.

BIRD RESCUE ASSOCIATION, Eastbourne Bird Hospital, 29 Arundel Road, Eastbourne, East Sussex BN21 2EG
Telephone: 0323 23875   Proprietor: Margaret King
Small bird hospital and sanctuary of many years' standing, with full veterinary support. Treatment of injured and oiled birds; rehabilitation or permanent sanctuary. Long-term aims are to see many bird hospitals throughout the country. Over 1,000 birds received annually; now trying to reduce intake but never refuses a bird in distress. Very willing to advise those who want to establish similar centres. Registered charity.

BIRD OF PREY RESCUE CENTRE, Crooked Meadow, Stidston
Lane, South Brent, Devon TQ10 9JS
Telephone: 03647 2174   Proprietor: Mrs J. E. L. Vinson
Mrs Vinson has been dealing specifically with sick and injured wild birds
of prey for about twenty years. Main object is to return as many as possible
to the wild: adults are returned to the exact territory where they were found
but hand-reared orphans are released from the centre. Sanctuary given to
permanently disabled birds. Indoor treatment pens; large outdoor aviaries and
release pens; close association with a veterinary hospital with particular interest
in wildlife rescue. Takes in casualties from RSPCA, RSPB, police and general
public. LRK.

BRENT LODGE BIRD AND WILDLIFE TRUST, Cow Lane,
Sidlesham, Chichester, West Sussex
Telephone: 024356 672   Proprietor: Dennis Fenter
The admirable Dennis Fenter previously ran a bird hospital at Eartham, and
is now backed by a supportive Trust at Sidlesham, where there is ample
outdoor space for raptors, seabirds and waterfowl (who have a large pond)
as well as indoor accommodation for sick birds and small mammals. Even
a sick swan can have half a barn to itself if necessary! Wide network of helpers
prepared to act as ambulance drivers etc. Full medical and surgical facilities.

CARE FOR THE WILD, 26 North Street, Horsham, West Sussex
RH12 1BN
Telephone: 0403 50557   Proprietor: Bill Jordan
Bill Jordan is the author of the classic wildlife rescue book, *Care of the Wild.*
Under the umbrella of the registered charity, Care for the Wild, he deals with
inquiries about sick and injured animals on a daily basis and gives first aid
to casualties. No facilities for fox-sized animals yet (though can pass them
on to other sanctuaries) but hoping to buy and equip own sanctuary and
would appreciate support from the public to this end. The aims of Care for
the Wild are simply to protect wildlife from cruelty, suffering and exploitation
and to educate the public on how this can be done, as well as helping sick
and injured wildlife either directly or by giving advice to the public.

GRAHAME DANGERFIELD WILDLIFE TRUST, Bowers Heath,
Harpenden, Hertfordshire AR5 5EE
Telephone: 05827 66229   Proprietor: Grahame Dangerfield
Grahame Dangerfield's wildlife trust is new in that it has only recently been
officially registered as a charity, but this naturalist has been running a Wildlife
Breeding Centre at Harpenden for many years, specialising in birds of prey
and wild cats and helped by Caroline Brown, an expert on the rearing of
young raptors. The centre also takes in all kinds of casualties brought by the

public—wild mammals as well as every kind of bird—and the centre now deals almost entirely with British wildlife casualties rather than breeding endangered species. There is a field station in Cornwall which cares for injured and orphaned Cornish wildlife. Although the Trust is in its formative stages at the time of writing, the Cornish scheme is well under way and will include a nature reserve in the Camel Valley in due course.

THE FALCONRY CENTRE, Newent, Gloucestershire GL18 1JJ
Telephone: 0531 820286   Proprietor: J. and J. Parry-Jones
There is nothing that the Parry-Jones centre does not know about birds of prey, and it leads the world in breeding them, with a collection of more than 200 birds on display. Flying demonstrations are given four times a day and visitors are very welcome. It is not a rescue centre for wildlife casualties but it is an invaluable source of information and advice, much of which can be gleaned from Jemima Parry-Jones's book, *Falconry—Care, Captive Breeding and Conservation.*

FERNE ANIMAL SANCTUARY, Wambrook, Chard, Somerset
Telephone: 04606 5214
Founded more than fifty years ago by the late Nina, Duchess of Hamilton and Brandon, this sanctuary was originally devoted to the pets that service people had to leave behind them during the Second World War. Today unwanted dogs, cats, horses and other domestic species still come to the sanctuary though space is limited and therefore many have to be turned away. Wildlife is not accepted as the RSPCA Wildlife Unit at Little Creech is only a few miles away. In the case of injured domestic animals, the advice is that they should be taken directly to a vet or the RSPCA, though the sanctuary will help if it can. Rehoming is carried out wherever possible. Work also includes helping children to understand the needs of animals. Registered charity.

THE HAWK CONSERVANCY, Weyhill, Andover, Hampshire
SP11 8DY
Telephone: 0264 772252   Proprietors: Mr and Mrs R. H. Smith
Not a rescue centre but run by falconers who know a great deal about birds of prey. Visitors welcome during the regular flying demonstrations.

HEAVEN'S GATE ANIMAL RESCUE CENTRE, West Henley,
Langport, Somerset TA10 9BE
Telephone: 0458 252656
Founded by Annabelle Walter in 1983 to help all types of domesticated species in any kind of trouble—unwanted pets, foals due to be slaughtered, battery hens, geese, cows, goats, horses, guinea-pigs, ducks and, of course, dogs and

cats. Space is limited (about 250 in residence at any one time) and no animal is put down unless it is incurably ill or incurably dangerous. Rehoming is the aim, once an animal has fully recovered. Please telephone before taking any animal to the centre to see if there is room for it, or whether the centre can suggest alternatives. If an injured animal is found, telephone Heaven's Gate immediately for advice. The centre does not have the facilities to look after wildlife. Registered charity.

HESSILHEAD WILDLIFE RESCUE TRUST, Gateside, Beith, Ayrshire KA15 1HT
Telephone: 05055 2415   Proprietors: Gay and Andrew Christie
In the late 1960s the Christies cared for an orphaned fox cub and gradually began to acquire experience of other wildlife species. By 1987 they were treating about 400 casualties a year and at that stage set up the Hessilhead Wildlife Rescue Trust. This excellent centre is based on a woodland smallholding in North Ayrshire and its aims are to rescue, repair and rehabilitate injured wildlife, and to rear orphaned creatures so that they can be returned to the wild. There is a small hospital building with veterinary support, and there are recuperation aviaries and release pens, with plans for even better facilities for waterfowl and deer. LRK. 24-hour rescue service, with volunteers running a courier service to collect injured creatures and orphans. In the interests of the casualties, visitors by appointment only. Registered charity, with adoption schemes by way of sponsorship.

THE HOME OF REST FOR HORSES, Westcroft Stables, Speen Farm, Aylesbury, Bucks HP19 0PP
Founded more than a hundred years ago (1886). Main aims are to enable the "poorer classes" to procure rest and skilled treatment for their animals when such care is needed; to provide a place of refuge for ponies and horses whose owners have been proved guilty of cruelty or neglect; and to provide a suitable asylum for a limited number of "Old Favourites" on reasonable terms. Equines only.

HYDESTILE WILDLIFE HOSPITAL, Nutwood Cottage, New Road, Hydestile, Godalming, Surrey
Proprietors: Graham and Lynn Cornick
Wildlife casualty centre run by an experienced couple who never turn an animal away but who find themselves overwhelmed by the numbers—they often find themselves taking in orphans which have grown too big and too expensive for other rescuers to maintain. Considerable knowledge of foxes, deer and squirrels in particular.

LOCKWOOD HOME OF REST FOR OLD AND SICK DONKEYS, Hatch Lane, Sandhills, Wormley, Godalming, Surrey
Telephone: 042879 2409   Proprietor: Mrs Kay Lockwood
A permanent home for donkeys: they are given sanctuary here for life. There are also old horses and a few ponies saved from the slaughterer, along with various goats, cats, dogs, pigs and poultry either saved or dumped on the doorstep. But the main reason for the sanctuary is to give old and sick donkeys a happier life. Open to visitors at all times.

MARINE LIFE AND WILDLIFE RESCUE, Newlands Estate, Bacton, Norfolk
Telephone: 0692 650540   Proprietor: Harry Nickerson
Run from Harold Nickerson's home for several years, this centre specialises in caring for oiled birds and distressed seals. Help of all kinds from the public is appreciated—finance of course (it is not a registered charity), lots of sprats and herrings for feeding the patients, and also representatives in coastal districts who can be trained to handle seals, birds and other wildlife casualties until they can be brought to Bacton for treatment. Harold Nickerson works in collaboration with Brenda Giles's seal rescue service at King's Lynn, and is a marine life conservationist.

MILLHOUSE ANIMAL SANCTUARY, Mayfield Road, Fulwood, Sheffield S10 4PR
Telephone: 0742 302907
A sanctuary for larger domesticated mammals in the Sheffield area—horses, ponies, donkeys, cows, sheep, pigs and goats. Will take in any of these species in distress—neglected, sick, rejected, confiscated by the RSPCA or simply unwanted or lost. Permanent home given to those that are not healthy enough to be given new, kind homes elsewhere under an adoption scheme by which the adopter guarantees that the animal will be cared for, given veterinary treatment when necessary, and returned to the sanctuary if no longer wanted. Alternatively, adopters can leave the animal in the sanctuary's care and sponsor its expenses. No animal is ever sold or given away, and only rarely is an animal not accepted. Those received in poor condition or injured are immediately treated and nursed; those that have no further prospects of a reasonable quality of life are humanely put to sleep. Millhouse is a sanctuary, not an animal hospital, but it will take in livestock which have been ill-treated.

MOUSEHOLE WILD BIRD HOSPITAL AND SANCTUARY ASSOCIATION LTD, Mousehole, Penzance, Cornwall TR19 6SR
Telephone: 0736 731386
Founded in 1928 by the Misses Yglesias, this sanctuary became famous during the Torrey Canyon disaster when it handled more than 8,000 oiled birds.

The RSPCA ran the hospital for about twenty years until it had to withdraw financial support in 1975 when funds were tight; a public appeal then produced enough finances and support for the hospital to continue, and it was registered as a charity in 1976. Its aims are to accept any bird in need of care, to heal it and to return it to the wild. Those which cannot be rehabilitated and which respond well to captivity are given sanctuary for the remainder of their lives; those beyond help are humanely destroyed. In a typical year 1,500 birds are treated.

NEWBURY WILDLIFE HOSPITAL AND REHABILITATION CENTRE, The Cemetery Lodge, Newtown, Newbury, Berkshire
Telephone: 0635 45009   Proprietors: Louise and Yvonne Veness
Accepts all species of wildlife casualties for care and rehabilitation.

NEW QUAY BIRD HOSPITAL, Penfoel, Cross Inn, Llandysul, Dyfed SA44 6NR
Telephone: 0545 560462   Proprietor: Alan Bryant
A well-known bird hospital with plenty of experience of oiled birds, including swans.

THE OTTER TRUST, Earsham, Bungay, Suffolk
Proprietor: Philip Wayre   Telephone: 0986 3470
A haven for otters covering 200 miles of unpolluted waterways and a centre on the banks of the river Waveney where captive otters are bred for reintroduction into the wild. Western branch at North Petherwin, Launceston, Cornwall. Will always advise on otter problems—and will no doubt advise strongly that any distressed or orphaned otter should be dealt with only by experts. The Trust also carries out detailed otter surveys and eco-system studies, and its education committee has set up a nature trail, produced literature for school-party visits, and developed a mobile interpretative centre emphasising the importance of wetlands conservation.

OWL RESCUE, Threxton, Watton, Norfolk
A voluntary group with a special interest in breed-and-release schemes. Takes in diurnal raptors and works with the Hawk Trust, the East Anglian Raptor Association and BOBARS to breed and release barn owls. Operates nationally and has travelled as far as Dorset and Kent to collect birds, but not on a regular basis—mainly to disperse birds from different bloodlines into new areas. Concentrates largely on the barn owl because of its endangered status but will take any species of birds of prey. Operates on a strictly non-buying/selling basis, and virtually all funding is from members' own pockets. LRK.

OWL SYMPOSIUM
The idea of owl expert Bernard Sayers, who saw the need for a forum for owl keepers and rescuers. First symposium in 1987; second in 1988. These

events are privately organised by Sayers but attract all the experts as well as large numbers of owl enthusiasts. The published papers (full of useful practical information) are on sale from 164 Chelmer Road, Chelmsford, Essex CM2 6AB. Although largely for keepers of captive owls, the information is also invaluable for rescuers and rehabilitators.

PINEWOOD OWL PARLIAMENT, Forest Glen, Longmoor Road, Liphook, Hampshire GU30 7PG
Telephone: 0428 725243   Proprietors: Ian and Valerie Brice
Barn owl breeding and rehabilitation, privately run by the Brices, who will also care for many other species of bird. Have successfully released more than 60 young barn owls into carefully selected habitats during the last six years or so. Have now set up a sponsorship scheme for captive-breeding barn owls in order to allow the release programme to continue and also sponsorship for injured owls unable to be rehabilitated. Useful report on some aspects of captive-breeding barn owls. LRK. Why "POP?" Believe it or not, a gathering of owls is known as a parliament.

RAPTOR REHABILITATION AND RESCUE CENTRE,
18 The Park, Hewell Grange, Redditch, Worcestershire B97 6QF
Proprietor: Steven Wyton
Rehabilitation unit for birds of prey, including breeding.

RAPTOR RESCUE, 38 Upper Clabdens, Ware, Herts SG12 7HB
Proprietor: Mike Abbey
Nationwide service for raptors.

SEA LIFE CENTRE, Barcaldine, Connel, Argyll PA37 1SE
Telephone: 063172 386
There are several Sea Life Centres, the concept for which was originated by John Mace, who practised as a vet for many years and was fascinated by marine wildlife. The Barcaldine centre was the first to open, in 1979: it is ten miles north of Oban and its displays manager, Laurance Larmour, has the dubious pleasure of dealing with all the "abandoned" seal pups people insist on picking up from the beaches.

    The Sea Life Centres are not designed as seal rescue centres: they are in effect marine zoos (though they would flinch at the description) where people can come and see resident seals and all sorts of marine fish at close quarters. However, because of their captive-seal breeding programme combined with the rearing of the wild "orphans" brought in for care, they have gained considerable knowledge with respect to the husbandry and nutrition needs of seals of all ages and are very willing to share that knowledge with competent seal rescuers; they are also willing to suggest good contacts for those who have any problems with seals. The other Sea Life Centres are at Weymouth, Dorset (Lodmoor Country Park) and Southsea, Hampshire (on the seafront at Clarence Esplanade) but these do not handle seals.

SEAL CENTRES
Some of the main seal centres, all of which are specialists, are shown below. For technical information, try the **Sea Mammal Research Unit** at Cambridge. If *you* find a sick seal, contact the local police or RSPCA/SSPCA.

Scotland
ISLAY AND JURA SEAL ACTION GROUP, Kildaton, Islay Telephone: 0496 2411
ISLE OF SKYE FIELD CENTRE, Broadford, Isle of Skye Telephone: 04712 487
LITTLE LINGA HOLM: Island sanctuary purchased by Ferne Animal Sanctuary, run by the Dunters (Orkney Environmental Concern Society). Orkney Mainland Telephone: 08567 3364
SSPCA OILED-BIRD CLEANING CENTRE, Middlebank Farm, Masterton Road, By Dunfermline, Fife

England
DOCKING SEAL RESCUE UNIT (RSPCA/Greenpeace) Fakenham, Norfolk Telephone: 04858 209
CORNWALL SEAL RESCUE (Ken Jones) Gweek, Helston, Cornwall
WEST NORFOLK SEAL RESCUE SERVICE (Brenda and Alan Giles), King's Lynn, Norfolk
NATURELAND (John Yeddon), Skegness

SURREY BIRD RESCUE AND CONSERVATION CENTRE,
Chertsey, Surrey
This is perhaps the longest established and largest rehabilitation centre in the south of England and is by no means limited to birds: they also work with wild mammals such as badgers, deer and hedgehogs, and have a number of successful breeding projects involving rescued and injured wildlife, including swans and tortoises. However, with 450 animals on the premises they are already very busy indeed and do not seek to increase their workload.

THREE OWLS BIRD SANCTUARY, Wolstenholme Fold, Norden,
Rochdale, Lancs OL11 5UD
Telephone: 0706 42162   Proprietor: Eileen J. Watkinson
Bird hospital founded in 1962. Provides a round-the-clock service for anyone finding a wild bird in distress. Owl barns, aviaries, 4-acre reserve for flying exercise before rehabilitation with wetland, woodland, meadowland and pools. Resident population of about 500 birds, with roughly 600 casualties taken

in each year. Experienced at hand-rearing fledglings. Small heronry based on disabled pair breeding free-flying birds. Visitors welcome Sunday afternoons, other times by arrangement. Registered charity.

VINCENT WILDLIFE TRUST, Baltic Exchange Buildings, 21 Bury Street, London EC3A 5AU
Trust ecologists: J. and R. Green, Barjarg, Barrhill, Girvan, Ayrshire KA26 0RB
Jim and Rosemary Green deal specifically with orphaned and injured otters in Ayrshire, returning the animals to the wild in collaboration with the NCC. Most distressed otters turn out to be young orphans, needing at least ten months in captivity under special conditions, and the Greens strongly advise that the animals should be passed on to them or to the Otter Trust as quickly as possible.

WEST WILLIAMSTON OILED BIRDS CENTRE, Lower House Farm, West Williamston, Kilgetty, S. Pembs SA68 0TL
Telephone: 06467 236   Warden: Mrs G. Hains
Centre run by the West Wales Nature Trust (WWNT). Can deal with very limited numbers of oiled birds at the centre (say, eight a day) but also acts as a holding facility for larger numbers of oiled birds which will be taken to the RSCPA unit at Little Creech in Somerset for cleaning and rehabilitation.

WILD BIRD RESCUE CENTRE, 10 Quarely Road, Havant, Hampshire PO9 4DU
Telephone: 0705 452521   Proprietor: Eileen Falconer
Family concern, supported by many volunteers (more than fifty voluntary "ambulance" drivers using their own cars). Takes in injured, sick and oiled wild birds, also small wild animals. All species of bird cared for, with veterinary support for badly injured.

ZOOS

Good zoos can be an excellent source of information for animal rescuers: they have a great deal of experience with nutrition, breeding, and rearing young animals. Some people have reservations or strong moral feelings about zoos but, in the interests of animal casualties, such qualms should perhaps be set aside for the sake of learning as much as possible in order to save lives and relieve distress in any animals which come into your care. Many are only too willing to help: for example, Bristol Zoo receives hundreds of calls a year from members of the public wondering what to do with an animal casualty, a wild orphan, an escaped exotic or a new pet. If you have a local zoo, there is no harm in asking. However, zoos are not casualty centres: it is not their role to take in sick, injured, orphaned or stray animals and indeed most of them would refuse to accept such animals for fear of introducing disease among their own captive stock.

Some zoos are much better than others, especially those with a genuine interest in conservation, and it is these that are the most likely to be willing to give advice when asked. London Zoo, in Regent's Park, has a substantial database and reference library with masses of information on subjects like the composition of different mammalian milks. Marwell Zoological Park near Winchester in Hampshire has an excellent reputation worldwide for its conservation work: it not only breeds endangered species in captivity but also takes steps to rehabilitate them in the wild in some instances (for example, Przewalski's horse, scimitar-horned oryx, Hartmann's mountain zebra). Jersey Zoological Park is another "conservation" zoo, and there are several others. Then there are the bird collections, where there is considerable expertise in hand-rearing various species. For information on any member of the pheasant family (which includes Britain's common pheasant, all the ornamental species, peacocks and the domestic hen, among others) contact the World Pheasant Association which is at the Child-Beale Wildlife Trust, Lower Basildon, Reading, Berkshire.

The following central organisations, each with very different attitudes towards zoos, are willing to give advice on useful contacts in specific cases.

Association of British Wild Animal Keepers
Contact: Mrs June Sherborne, Editor of *Ratel,* 12 Tackley Road, Eastville, Bristol BS5 6UQ
Most of the members of ABWAK are employed in zoos, wildlife parks etc., and they share their detailed practical knowledge through their bi-monthly magazine, *Ratel.* Its editor will give advice or be able to pass an enquiry to another ABWAK member if necessary or appropriate, but she would be grateful if enquirers would enclose a stamped, self-addressed envelope.

Zoo Check, Cherry Tree Cottage, Coldharbour, Dorking, Surrey RH5 6HA
Telephone: 0306 712091
Zoo Check's aims are to check and prevent all types of abuse to captive animals and wildlife, to phase out zoos and (where appropriate) support conservation centres, to promote international support for the conservation of animals in their natural habitat, to end the taking of animals from the wild, and to encourage respect for the natural world and an understanding of its interrelationships. It is a charitable trust with many consultants, each specialising in particular problems with particular species, and many veterinary surgeons who help with difficult cases, especially abroad. If you have a special problem, Zoo Check might be able to point you in the right direction.

Zoological Society of London, Regent's Park, London NW1 4RY
Founded by Sir Stamford Raffles for "the advancement of Zoology and
Animal Physiology, and the introduction of new and curious subjects of the
Animal Kingdom". Granted five acres of land in Regent's Park to open
London Zoo in 1828. Very important central source of information on all
aspects of wild animal husbandry, including veterinary side, for native as well
as exotic species.

APPENDIX 1

PROCEDURE FOR CLEANING AND
REHABILITATING OILED BIRDS

(Rescuers should read the section on 'Oil and Pollution' in Chapter 4 before attempting to clean an oiled bird. Even then, it is still best left to the experts.)

(a) The bird will almost certainly be suffering from enteritis on top of shock, and needs dosing with something like Kaobiotic tablets for up to a maximum of seven days, or until it is ready to be washed if that is sooner. The tablets counteract the effects of ingested oil. However, they are antibiotic and should be respected as such: do not give them (or any other antibiotics) during the week before a bird's release.

(b) The bird needs to eat; it will have been unable to do so adequately since it began to suffer the effects of pollution and will therefore be in a weakened state, which does not enhance its prospects for recovery. If necessary, it will have to be force-fed. In these early stages it is probably best to stick to raw strips of filleted white fish (for example, plaice, sole, cod and whiting) for seabirds rather than give whole fish whose bones might aggravate internal inflammations caused by the effects of ingested oil. Force-feeding is bound to be stressful and should not become a routine.

(c) Assess the bird's chances of recovery. This might not be a priority if you are only dealing with a couple of birds but if larger numbers are involved it is much better to concentrate on potential survivors than to spread your resources over all of them and risk losing the lot. Even with a crowd of birds, it is important to consider each of them as an individual, which means you need to be able to recognise each one and monitor it separately. For this reason it is better to keep seabirds in pairs in cages, with some form of identification, rather than have them all loose together in a room. They will feel more secure in their cages anyway: loose birds tend to panic when someone enters the room, and there is also a considerable problem with keeping the floor clean and avoiding foot ailments if the floor is of concrete.

The assessment should of course include any sign of external injuries but perhaps more important are: a general air of alertness; a nicely rounded bright eye; a tendency to be aggressive (if the bird makes at least some attempt to escape from its box, so much the better: it has the will to live—as long as it does not become frantic); a lack of obvious physical disabilities which would make the bird less viable; a degree of plumpness on either side of the breastbone (sternum); an ability to walk with a gait natural to the species, and a natural way of holding its wings close to its body. Ignore the degree of oiling: it is the fitness of the bird itself that counts and quite often the oiliest bird is fitter than one which has only a patch of oil on it. Birds with oil in their faeces and significant traces of oil in the mouth are not the most promising candidates.

Adverse pointers include glazed eyes, a tendency to lie down with the rump and lower back pronouncedly arched (which means there are internal problems), an inability to stand properly on its webs, or a general lack of condition and bodyweight.

(d) Do not attempt to clean a bird yourself unless you have *all* the following facilities:

- Enough hot water (at 40–42 °C) with high enough pressure and consistency of pressure to be sprayed *continuously* at a constant rate of flow for at least an hour for each bird.
- A large sink or bath.
- An ample supply of washing-up liquid, preferably a cheaper type and specifically Co-op Green or Winfield (for good, proven reasons—the cheaper ones are more effective than the thicker, more expensive ones, nor do they harm the bird's eyes) and lots of newspaper.
- Ample storage for frozen food.
- Two people—one to hold the bird while the other washes it—and at least one of them

227

with appropriate training.

● The ability and application to be absolutely meticulous and thorough throughout the whole procedure, and plenty of uninterrupted time to be so.

● A warm, very clean room (no dust or cobwebs) or large clean pen where the washed birds can preen and rest and where the ambient temperature can be maintained at a constant 17 °C.

● An easily-cleaned pool with a constant waterflow through it, for testing plumage quality before a bird is released.

● For ducks, geese and swans, a dry outdoor recovery pen, preferably on good turf and with alternative pens to be used in rotation, where the birds can convalesce for up to three months and can "weather off" certain oils which are resistant to the washing process.

(e) Seabirds need to be returned to their environment as quickly as possible and therefore the cleaning methods need to be intensive. The whole process can take, say, one-and-a-half to two hours to clean one guillemot-sized bird, followed by an overnight stay in a warm room for preening, then a series of waterproofing and buoyancy tests over several days until the plumage is proven to be in perfect condition for release.

(f) Inland waterfowl are often affected by different kinds of oil which cannot be removed by the washing process. They therefore need to be given a secure, *dry* outdoor pen for as long as it takes for the oil to weather off, and that could be as much as three months of feeding, watching and protecting from predators, and in due course adequate exercise to ensure their muscles are fit enough for the wild. They should not be allowed to bathe during the weathering process but must be able to get their heads underwater.

(g) To clean oiled seabirds, follow these procedures scrupulously and never take any short cuts or half measures:

(i) In a sink of hot water (42 °C—you can only just bear to put your hand into it) make up a solution of 2 parts washing-up liquid to 100 parts water—say, half a cup of washing-up liquid to a large washing-up bowl.

(ii) Restrain the bird's bill with an elastic band for your own protection, but make sure its nostrils are not impeded. Be prepared to remove the band immediately if any vomiting or distress is evident.

(iii) Immerse the bird up to its neck in the solution.

(iv) Work the solution very thoroughly through the plumage in order to remove absolutely every trace of oil. Work methodically and always in the same sequence to make sure nothing is missed. Start with the head (even if it does not seem to be oily) and neck, then the back, the top of the tail, the top of the right wing, the top of the left wing. Do not be too gentle: feathers are quite tough as long as you avoid breaking the actual shaft, which is especially important on a flight feather, so be sensibly thorough on the back and wings.

(v) Now turn the bird over (which it will not like at all) and work on the breast, then the abdomen, then around the vent area, under the tail, along the right flank and under the right wing, then along the left flank and under the left wing. Be particularly thorough, cleaning every last tiny feather on the underside, right down to the skin, because this is the part of a seabird which will always be in the water in future.

(vi) Change the solution at intervals so that it remains effective and as near 42 °C as possible all the time. Give the bird a quick rinse with hot water (42 °C) between each change of the solution.

(vii) Remove *all* traces of the detergent from the bird, using a hand-held spray of hot water (42 °C) under high pressure with a concentrated jet. Have the bird held so that the rinsed-off residues flow away from plumage which has already been sprayed, and jet the water *against* the natural lie of the feathers so that it gets right through to the skin. Work methodically as before. Make sure that your own hands (and the holder's) are thoroughly sluiced before touching a rinsed part of the bird. Keep on spraying *until the water forms beads* on the surface of the feathers—a sign that the detergent has been removed and the feathers are back to normal, which means they will be virtually dry. The whole appearance of the feathers at this stage should look dry, except perhaps the tail and wings of a cormorant or shag. This rinsing process is absolutely vital; a bird's buoyancy can be destroyed if there is the slightest trace of cleaning agent still on any feather, and that would be disastrous when the bird is released.

(viii) As soon as a bird is clean, you must be very careful to touch it only with very clean hands (free of sweat and oil). Do not dry the bird artificially with towels or cloths: the slightest trace of detergent on them could destroy all the waterproofing you have just so laboriously achieved, and anyway the bird will be naturally virtually dry if your work has been thorough.

(ix) Put the bird in a warm, dry, clean room to preen and rest. Have clean paper on the floor but do not use newspaper unless you can get clean, ink-free "end rolls" from a printer. Try paper tablecloths or kitchen paper. Make sure appropriate food is available for the bird, which will by now be ravenous—perhaps with relief. Use a fan heater if necessary to take the chill off the room and achieve a uniform 17 °C. Remember to remove the elastic band from the bird's beak, and then leave it in the warmth and dark in complete peace and privacy all night to rest. Do not restrain or confine it: give it the freedom of the floor.

(x) The next morning, the bird will want and need to bathe itself, out of doors in a very clean pool which is not contaminated by faeces or bits of food. Once the bird has been allowed access to bathing, it must thereafter have constant access at its own volition. The pools should be about 12 inches deep and must be cleaned out completely every day, even if they are constantly sluiced by running water. Do not throw fish into the water: that would produce an oil film on the pool and probably wreck the feathers' waterproofing all over again. Give food in a separate water-bowl. Provide a limited standing area against a false "cliff" face.

(xi) Watch the bird discreetly to see that it is fit and remains buoyant; if it does not, your washing and rinsing were not thorough. Then try the final test to see if the bird is ready for rehabilitation. Keep it on the pool for at least thirty minutes consecutively, then examine it very closely to see that it is completely dry. If there is even the tiniest damp patch on the plumage (excepting the tail and wings of a shag) do *not* release the bird because it will perish. A sure sign of trouble is if the bird feels unbalanced on the water and flaps its wings to regain stability.

(xii) When the bird does pass the final test and is plump and generally fit, have it ringed by a qualified British Trust for Ornithology ringer (telephone 044282 3461 for your nearest one) then get advice from the local coastguard, nature reserve warden or local fishermen about a suitable release site for the species and time of year. The site needs to be undisturbed and of course oil-free! Take the bird close to the shore and let it swim away (don't throw it over a cliff into mid-air). Watch its progress for a while: if it returns to the shore, it is not ready for release. Choose a reasonably calm day.

APPENDIX 2

PHYSICAL METHODS OF KIND KILLING

In most cases the kindest killing is by a veterinary surgeon, usually with an overdose of anaesthetic or gassing, except in the case of large livestock which are usually shot (either with a humane weapon such as a captive-bolt or free bullet pistol, or with a firearm used by an expert marksman). Fuller details of the physical methods suggested here are given in Chapter 5. Casualties can be divided broadly into groups according to the recommended methods of kind killing.

GROUP 1

- DOMESTIC AND LARGE WILD MAMMALS (cat, cattle, deer, dog, donkey, goat, horse, mule, pig, sheep)
- MARINE MAMMALS (dolphin, porpoise, seal, whale)

1ST METHOD: Captive-bolt or free bullet
2ND METHOD: Shooting (rifle or shotgun as appropriate)

GROUP 2

- WILD MAMMALS—CARNIVORES, LAGOMORPHS AND HEDGEHOGS (badger, ferret, fox, hare, hedgehog, mink, otter, pine marten, polecat, rabbit, stoat, weasel)
- GAMEBIRDS AND WATERFOWL

1ST METHOD: Shooting (rifle or shotgun as appropriate)
2ND METHOD: Stun/kill (or neck-break for lagomorphs and birds)

GROUP 3

- RODENTS AND SMALLER INSECTIVOROUS MAMMALS (dormouse, gerbil, guinea-pig, hamster, mole, mouse, rat, shrew, squirrel, vole)
- DOMESTIC POULTRY
- CAGE BIRDS AND MOST WILD BIRDS
- AMPHIBIANS, REPTILES AND FISH (Stun/kill)

Stun/kill or neck-break

GROUP 4

- INVERTEBRATES

Boil, freeze or crush

APPENDIX 3

NATURAL FOOD PREFERENCES
AND SUITABLE ALTERNATIVES

BIRDS: NATURAL FOOD PREFERENCES

Birds of Prey Most diurnal raptors take birds and rodents, but kestrels concentrate on small rodents, peregrines usually take only birds, and ospreys are specialist fish-eaters. Buzzards and eagles will take small rabbits; several species supplement their diets with insects, worms and frogs; and the golden eagle and kite will eat carrion. The owls generally hunt rodents, small birds and insects.

Corvids Apart from choughs (which favour insects) corvids will take eggs, insects, grubs, worms, small birds and mammals, seeds and grains, nuts, berries and fruit. Ravens and hooded crows will eat crustaceans and molluscs and, like carrion crows, they also scavenge carrion.

Seairds All this group prefer freshly caught fish. Terns, petrels and shearwaters like their fish small and also eat crustaceans. Eggs, carrion and small birds are taken by skuas and also by gulls, which will eat almost anything they can find.

Waders Most waders eat insects, grubs, worms, snails, molluscs, shellfish, shrimps, frogs, sandhoppers and sandworms. Some might also take mice or eat seaweed.

Inland Waterbirds Grebes, herons, bitterns and kingfishers take fish and most also eat frogs, tadpoles and insects. Grebes will eat crustaceans and shellfish; herons steal young waterfowl and water voles. Spoonbills prefer water plants but also fish and insects. Dippers like aquatic insects, larvae, water snails and frogs. The rails eat insects, worms, tadpoles, spawn, molluscs, berries, seeds, slugs, snails and shellfish; coots also eat grain and aquatic weeds.

Wildfowl Ducks' feeding habits vary according to species and in general they eat insects, worms, slugs, snails, shellfish, frogs, grain, berries, crustaceans and aquatic plants. Smew, mergansers and goosanders prefer fish, shellfish and crustaceans; shelduck also eat sandworms, sandhoppers, snails and seaweed. Swans eat aquatic plants, shellfish and insects but geese are land-grazers of grass, vegetation and grain.

Gamebirds, Poultry, Pigeons and Doves All these are mainly grain and seed eaters, but enjoy a wide variety of food including leaves, shoots, berries, nuts, caterpillars and insects.

Thrush Family and Starlings Thrushes, blackbirds, robins, chats, nightingales and starlings eat insects, grubs, earthworms, slugs, snails, fruit and berries.

Insectivores This large group includes birds which catch insects on the wing (swallows, swifts, martins, flycatchers) and a wide range of species feeding mainly on insects at various stages of their life cycle (e.g. caterpillars and grubs). Other insectivores such as many tits, woodpeckers, warblers, pipits and larks also eat berries, nuts and fruit or seeds and shoots.

Finches This stubby-beaked group also eats insects but their main food is seeds of various sizes, including in some cases grains, nuts and berries.

SUITABLE ALTERNATIVE FOODS FOR CAPTIVE BIRDS

Birds of Prey Day-old hatchery chicks, pinkies, RTA victims. Or strips of raw meat with supplements and roughage. Also livefood (mealworms, grasshoppers etc) for merlins, hawks and kites.

Corvids Minced raw meat with supplements, day-old chicks, RTA victims, plus choice of fruit, nuts, grubs, eggs, livefood.

Seabirds Essentially very fresh fish—sprats, whitebait, herring, strips of raw white fish (cod), freshwater shrimps—offered in shallow dish of water. Might need supplementary salt.

Waders Fresh fish in water; fresh shrimps, boiled rice, hard-boiled egg, minced meat, tinned salmon, livefood—all offered moist. Clams for oystercatchers. Do not watch or they will not feed. Many will only feed out-of-doors.

Water Birds Fresh fish (live minnows in water for kingfishers), mealworms, minced meat. Try more variety for rails—including tinned dogmeat, egg, bread, seeds, greens.

Wildfowl For ducks and swans, all food should be moist. Food for swans *must* be in or floating on water—fresh grass clippings, hydroponic grass, supplemented with chopped greens, lettuce, grain, soaked cornflakes, daily slice of bread, pondweed, grit. For ducks, offer food with shallow water container for dunking: soaked grain, duckweed, hydroponic grass, greens, chopped sprats, tinned dogmeat. Geese eat on dry land—turf of grass or hydroponic grass for grazing, with greens, grain, bread and grit.

Gamebirds, Poultry, Pigeons Grain or poultry feeds given on ground, with gizzard grit; also greens, animal protein (tinned dogmeat, Sluis, mealworms, grasshoppers etc.) and choice of fruit, berries, nuts, insects, brown bread, chopped egg.

Thrush family Earthworms in box of soil; mealworms, crickets, flies and other insects; ox-heart, snails, cheese, Sluis, berries, fruit, soaked raisins. Starlings similar but would prefer minced meat rather than earthworms.

Insectivores Insectivore mix (Sluis etc.) or minced meat with supplements, tinned dogmeat, steamed fish—decorate with token live mealworm to stimulate interest; egg, dried flies, grubs, millet, boiled rice. Swallows, swifts and martins difficult but house martins love mealworms (and termites!). For warblers, set up an insect trap for fresh insects or hang an attracting light bulb above the accommodation, or breed fruitflies.

Woodpeckers and Nuthatches Try hiding food in bark crevices—beef suet, nuts, fruit, egg, seeds, mealworms, grubs, sunflower seeds, grated cheese, shredded shrimps, insectivore mix—or smear peanut butter on bark. Nectar of honey in water.

Finches Wide range according to species. Basic avicultural finch mixes; add larger seeds for stronger billed, and richer for goldfinches and linnets (including hemp). Also wild foods according to species and season: tree seeds, leaf/flower buds, seedheads, weed seeds. Crushed peanuts in moderation. Daily fruit for many species, especially berries and dessert apple.

MAMMALS: NATURAL FOOD PREFERENCES

Carnivores Foxes are opportunists and take what is locally available and easiest by predation and scavenging: rabbits, rodents; earthworms, beetles; discarded livestock afterbirth, edible refuse, carrion; poultry and other birds; fruit and berries. Badgers are omnivorous: earthworms for preference but will also eat same as fox plus slugs, snails, amphibians, wasp grubs, grass, clover, grains. Mink take what they can: young rabbits, voles, rats, fish, water birds, crayfish, occasionally poultry and gamebirds. Otters eat mostly fish, crustaceans, amphibians, worms and a few insects. Other mustelids are efficient carnivores taking a wide variety of prey: small mammals, birds, frogs, lizards, insect larvae, earthworms, beetles, eggs, some carrion, possibly fish.

Insectivores Bats take all kinds of flying insects and also whisk small insects and spiders off foliage. Hedgehogs eat beetles, caterpillars, earthworms, flies, centipedes, spiders, slugs; occasionally eggs, carrion, fruit. Moles live largely on earthworms and insect larvae, also slugs, centipedes, millipedes. Shrews eat earthworms and beetles, also insects, spiders, snails, slugs, centipedes, woodlice. Water shrews also take small fish and amphibians; white-toothed species also take lizards, small rodents, and will eat fresh fish, meat and grain in captivity.

Rodents Mice eat a wide range, according to species and availability: fruits, nuts, grain, buds, seedlings, tree seeds, snails, arthropods, fungi, moss, bark, galls, dead leaves, earthworms. Harvest mice also take insects; dormice eat mostly nuts, fruit and berries, sunflower seeds, but not grain, though possibly buds and insects in spring; fat dormice sometimes eat apples, eggs and nestlings; house mice eat just about anything including plaster, soap, candles and glue! Rats are omnivores with preference for protein-rich and starch-rich foods such as cereals but will also eat meat, fish, bones, root crops, brassicas, weed seeds, earthworms, crustaceans, fruit and nuts. Voles are herbivorous but occasionally take insect larvae; water voles prefer aquatic plants and grasses, and might sample a dead fish. Squirrels have catholic tastes: tree seeds, nuts, foliage, buds, catkin pollen, sap; occasionally eggs, nestlings, small birds, insects and grubs; berries, roots, bulbs and seeds; also soil for minerals and roughage. Rabbits and hares eat a wide range of plant matter: grasses, crops (cereal, root, horticultural), young trees and bark, herbaceous plants, ling etc., and ingest own pellets to recycle nutrients.

Ungulates Cattle are grazers, especially of pasture, but also browse some leaves. Sheep are close-grazing ruminants, commonly eating grasses though in some places they eat seaweed or heath. Horses are essentially grazers but less efficient than ruminants at digesting grasses (their main source of nutrition). Deer graze and browse: grasses, sedges and rushes, shrubbery, herbs, lichens, ferns, fungi, bark, nuts, fruit and berries, brambles, ivy, flowers, heather; Chinese water deer also eat vegetables and root crops. Pigs are omnivorous: in the wild they eat roots, acorns, chestnuts, beechmast, plant stems, fungi, grain, insect larvae, earthworms, eggs, frogs, reptiles, carrion.

Marine Mammals Dolphins and porpoises are fish-eaters (herring, cod, whiting, sole, mackerel, pilchard) and also eat cuttlefish, octopus and crustaceans. The large toothless baleen whales strain planktonic animals from the seawater; some also take fish as big as herring. The toothed whales eat squid, cuttlefish, fish like herring and cod, and perhaps crustaceans, while killer whales take other marine mammals, penguins and large fish. Seals eat mainly fish and the young take quite a lot of shrimps; grey seals also eat cuttlefish and whelks. Walruses feed almost exclusively on clams but might develop a taste for young seals.

SUITABLE ALTERNATIVE FOODS FOR CAPTIVE MAMMALS

Carnivores For badgers and foxes: tinned dogfood and dog biscuits, whole raw egg, pinkies, day-old chicks, RTA victims, earthworms, beetles, choice of fruit. (If jaw is broken, offer meaty soups, milk, baby cereal, Complan, Farex.) Otters: fish, eels, frogs, newts, mice, rabbits, crabs, day-old chicks, minced raw meat with supplements. Other mustelids: day-old chicks, RTA victims, rodents (need whole carcases perhaps three times a week if fed mainly on raw meat or tinned food, and occasional treat of raw egg and milk).

Insectivores Bats: give water before first feed, then liquid diet (squeezed mealworms) and eventually live insects if possible or dampened dried flies, mashed egg, tinned catfood, finely ground liver (tinned dogfood or scrambled egg in emergency). Hedgehogs: Sluis Universal, earthworms, minced raw meat with supplements, mushy tinned dogfood, chicken, liver, offal, pilchards, dead mouse, cottage cheese, raw or cooked egg, slugs and snails, peanuts, occasional biscuit; no bread-and-milk but plenty of drinking water. Moles: earthworms in a box of soil; could try tinned dogfood; need constant access to food. Shrews: insects, woodlice, snails, earthworms, tinned dogfood—constant access (they die of starvation within hours).

Rodents Grain, chickenfeed, nuts, acorns, clover and dandelion leaves and flowers; lots of vegetation for water vole (reeds, iris leaves, grasses); choice of seeds and grains for harvest mouse (also loves brown bread); plenty of drinking water or moist fruit and vegetables. Squirrels: choice of unsalted nuts in shell; choice of seasonal berries, fruit, seeds, greenstuffs, cereals, grain, poultry pellets—prefers to eat little and often (for invalids, use standard invalid foods in liquid form given by pipette at first). Rabbits and hares: assorted herbage, e.g. leaves from grasses, dandelion, clover, green vegetables, lettuce, carrot and turnip tops; cereals, hay, apples, pet-shop rabbit food.

Ungulates Fresh grazing if possible, or freshly cut grass—deer also need access to soil for minerals (chunk of turf), a little ivy to stimulate appetite, brambles or rose shoots and flowers.

Deer and domesticated livestock also like sweet hay, root and leaf vegetables, foliage from broadleaf trees, nuts (including peanuts), cattle/deer pellets.

Marine Mammals Offer adult seals whole fish, or fish soup for young—best left to the experts. Do not even try to feed cetaceans.

APPENDIX 4

PROTECTED SPECIES UNDER THE WILDLIFE AND COUNTRYSIDE ACT, 1981 (revised 1986)

BIRDS

ALL BIRDS, except those listed in Schedule 1, Part II, and in Schedule 2, are fully protected throughout the year, including their nests and eggs.

SCHEDULE 1, PART I Birds protected by special penalties at all times. (* = also SCHEDULE 4 species; must be registered if kept in captivity. Schedule 4 includes all birds of prey except Old World vultures and many other birds as shown here.)

*Avocet	*Greenshank	*Sandpiper, Wood
*Bee-eater	Gull, Little	Scaup
*Bittern	Gull, Mediterranean	*Scoter, Common
*Bittern, Little	*Harriers (all)	*Scoter, Velvet
*Bluethroat	*Heron, Purple	*Serin
Brambling	*Hobby	*Shorelark
*Bunting, Cirl	*Hoopoe	*Shrike, Red-backed
*Bunting, Lapland	*Kingfisher	*Spoonbill
*Bunting, Snow	*Kite, Red	*Stilt, Black-winged
*Buzzard, Honey	*Merlin	*Stint, Temminck's
*Chough	*Oriole, Golden	Swan, Bewick's
*Corncrake	*Osprey	Swan, Whooper
*Crake, Spotted	Owl, Barn	*Tern, Black
*Crossbills (all)	Owl, Snowy	*Tern, Little
*Curlew, Stone	*Peregrine	*Tern, Roseate
*Divers (all)	*Petrel, Leach's	*Tit, Bearded
*Dotterel	*Phalarope,	*Tit, Crested
*Duck, Long-tailed	Red-necked	*Treecreeper,
*Eagle, Golden	*Plover, Kentish	Short-toed
*Eagle, White-tailed	*Plover,	*Warbler, Cetti's
*Falcon, Gyr	Little Ringed	*Warbler, Dartford
*Fieldfare	*Quail, Common	*Warbler, Marsh
*Firecrest	*Redstart, Black	*Warbler, Savi's
Garganey	*Redwing	*Whimbrel
*Godwit, Black-tailed	*Rosefinch, Scarlet	*Woodlark
*Goshawk	*Ruff	*Wryneck
*Grebe, Black-necked	*Sandpiper, Green	
*Grebe, Slavonian	*Sandpiper, Purple	

SCHEDULE 1, PART II Birds protected by special penalties during the close season (1st February to 31st August, or 21st February to 31st August below high-water mark) but may be killed or taken outside this period.

Goldeneye
Goose, Greylag (in Outer Hebrides, Caithness, Sutherland
and Wester Ross only)
Pintail

SCHEDULE 2, PART I Birds protected during the close season but may be killed or taken outside this period.

Capercaillie	Goose, Canada
Coot	Goose, Greylag
Duck, Tufted	Goose, Pink-footed
Gadwall	Goose, White-fronted
Goldeneye	Mallard

Moorhen	Snipe, Common
Pintail	Teal
Plover, Golden	Wigeon
Pochard	Woodcock
Shoveler	

SCHEDULE 2, PART II   Birds which may be killed or taken by authorised persons at all times.

Crow	Gull, Herring	Sparrow, House
Dove, Collared	Jackdaw	Starling
Gull, Great	Jay	Woodpigeon
Black-backed	Magpie	
Gull, Lesser	Pigeon, Feral	
Black-backed	Rook	

SCHEDULE 3, PART I   Birds which may be sold alive at all times if ringed and bred in captivity.

Blackbird	Greenfinch	Siskin
Brambling	Jackdaw	Starling
Bullfinch	Jay	Thrush, Song
Bunting, Reed	Linnet	Twite
Chaffinch	Magpie	Yellowhammer
Dunnock	Owl, Barn	
Goldfinch	Redpoll	

SCHEDULE 3, PART II   Birds which may be sold dead at all times.

Pigeon, Feral
Woodpigeon

SCHEDULE 3, PART III   Birds which may be sold dead from 1st September to 28th February.

Capercaillie	Pintail	Snipe, Common
Coot	Plover, Golden	Teal
Duck, Tufted	Pochard	Wigeon
Mallard	Shoveler	Woodcock

OTHER ANIMALS

SCHEDULE 5   It is normally an offence to kill, injure, take, possess or sell any of the following animals, whether alive or dead, or to disturb their place of shelter and protection or to destroy that place.

Adder (sale only)	Otter
Bats (all species)	Porpoises
Wild Cat	Slow-worm
Dolphins	Grass Snake
Dormouse	Smooth Snake
Common Frog (sale only)	Red Squirrel
Sand Lizard	Common Toad (sale only)
Viviparous Lizard	Natterjack Toad
Pine Marten	Marine Turtles
Great Crested or Warty Newt	Walrus
Palmate Newt (sale only)	Whales
Smooth Newt (sale only)	

(Also several insects, marine creatures etc.)

APPENDIX 5

USEFUL ADDRESSES

British Hedgehog Preservation Society, Knowbury House, Knowbury, Ludlow, Shropshire SY8 3LQ

British Herpetological Society, c/o Zoological Society of London, Regent's Park, London NW1 4RY

British Small Animals Veterinary Association, 5 St George's Terrace, Cheltenham, Glos GL50 3PT

Department of the Environment, Wildlife and Conservation Section, Tollgate House, Houlton Street, Bristol BS2 9DJ Telephone: 0272 218811 (for registration of birds of prey etc.)

Farming & Wildlife Trust, National Agricultural Centre, Stoneleigh, Kenilworth, Warks

Flora & Fauna Preservation Society, c/o Zoological Society of London, Regent's Park, London NW1 4RY

Forestry Commission, Wildlife Branch, Alice Holt Lodge, Wrecclesham, Farnham, Surrey GU10 4LH

Game Conservancy, Fordingbridge, Hants SP6 1EF

Institute of Terrestrial Ecology, Monks Wood Experimental Station, Abbots Ripton, Huntingdon, Camb PE17 2LS

Mammal Society, Burlington House, Piccadilly, London W1N 0LQ

National Dog Owners' Association, 39 North Road, Islington, London N7 9DP (for details of breed rescue centres)

Nature Conservancy Council, Northminster House, Peterborough, Cambs PE1 1UA *or* Hope Terrace, Edinburgh EH9 2AS

National Federation of Zoological Gardens, Zoological Gardens, Regent's Park, London NW1 4RT

Rare Breed Survival Trust, National Agriculture Centre, Kenilworth, Warwicks CV8 2LJ

Sea Mammals Research Unit, c/o British Antarctic Survey, High Cross, Madingley Road, Cambs CB3 0ET

Wildlife Disease Association, PO Box 886, Ames, Iowa 50010, USA

World Pheasant Association, Church Farm, Lower Basildon, Reading, Berks RG8 9PF

Zoological Society of London, Centre for Life Studies, Regent's Park, London NW1 4RY (advice on exotic animals).

APPENDIX 6

SUPPLIERS

Beecham Animal Health, Beecham House, Brentford, Middlesex TW8 9BD   (Lectade oral rehydration fluid)

Bioserve Inc., PO Box 450, Frenchtown, New Jersey, USA   (Primilac)

Birdquest International, 20 Lancaster Avenue, Besses o' the Barn, Whitefield, Manchester M25 6DE   (Claus insectivorous food; Livefoods—mealworms, crickets, locusts, fruitflies, wax moths; additives)

British Denkavit, Patrick House, West Quay Road, Poole, Dorset BH15 1JF   (Denkapup)

Championship Foods Ltd, Orwell, Royston, Herts SG8 5QX   (Horsepower)

E. W. Coombs Ltd, 25 Frindsbury Road, Strood, Kent ME2 4SU   (Sluis insectivorous food; Livefoods—mealworms, crickets)

Farley Health Products, Thane Road West, Nottingham NG2 3AA   (Complan, Farex, Casilan milk-derived protein supplement, Glucodin dextrose and vitamin C milk-free carbohydrate supplement, Ostermilk)

John E. Haith Ltd, Park Street, Cleethorpes, S. Humberside DN35 7PQ   (All types of bird food for all species)

Edric Higginbottom Laboratory Livefoods, High Bradfield, Sheffield S6 6LJ   (Livefoods—mealworms, crickets, locusts, fruitflies etc.)

Hoechst U.K. Ltd, PO Box 18, Hounslow, Middlesex TW4 6JH   (Cimicat, Welpi)

Intervet Laboratories Ltd, Science Park, Milton Road, Cambridge CB4 4BH   (SA37 supplement)

Mazuri Zoo Foods, Special Diet Service Ltd, PO Box 705, Witham, Essex CM8 3AD   (Special diets for wide range of zoo species, not usually able to supply in small quantities but considerable dietary expertise and could be helpful as reference point)

M.D. Components, Hamelin House, 211-213 Hightown Road, Luton, Beds L82 0VZ   (Animal handling equipment also a consultancy service on all animal control matters)

The Mealworm Company, Unit 1, Universal Crescent, North Anston Trading Estate, Sheffield S31 7JJ   (Livefood—O.C. additives)

Millpledge Pharmaceuticals Ltd, Whinleys Estate, Church Lane, Clarborough, Retford, Notts DN22 9NA   (Vet-amin multi-vitamin supplement; Can-addase enzyme supplement)

Milupa Ltd, Uxbridge Road, Hillingdon, Uxbridge UB10 0NE   (Milupa Infant Dessert—useful for fruit-eater baby birds)

Parke-Davis Veterinary, Usk Road, Pontypool, Gwent NP4 0YH   (Abidec multi-vitamin supplement)

Pedigree Petfoods, Waltham-on-the-Wolds, Melton Mowbray, Leics LE14 4RS   (Chum dogfood etc.; Trill birdseed)

Pet-AG Inc. and Borden Inc. Pet/Vet Products, 30W432 Rt. 20 Elgin, Illinois 60120, USA   (Esbilac, KMR, Multi-Milk)

Pet-Chef Health Products, Skates Lane, Sutton-on-Forest, York YO6 1HB   (Range of products for birds and pets)

Roche Products Ltd, Broadwater Road, Welwyn Garden City, Herts   (Vit D3 powder)

Shirley's, Ashe Laboratories Ltd, Leatherhead, Surrey   (Lactol)

E.R. Squibb & Sons Ltd, 141/149 Staines Road, Hounslow, Middlesex TW3 3JB   (Vionate multi-vitamin supplement)

Temple Cox Development Co. Ltd, Cray Avenue, Orpington, Kent BR5 3TT   (Animal graspers, nets etc.)

Uno Roestvastaal BV, Postbus 15, 6900 AA Zevenaar, Netherlands   (Ketch-All animal handling poles—obtainable from M.D. COMPONENTS)

Veterinary Drug Co. Plc, Common Road, Dunnington, Yorkshire YO1 5RU   (Dextrose powder)

Volac Feeds Ltd, Killeshandra, Co. Cavan   (Lamlac, Litterlac, Volac, Faramate)

W.A.M., Warren Farm Cottage, Headley Lane, Mickleham, Dorking, Surrey RH5 6DG   (Semark humane gamebird despatcher)

Wundpets, Unit G, Hadleigh Road Industrial Estate, Ipswich, Suffolk   (Bogena additives and insectivorous foods)

Wyeth Nutrition, Wyeth Laboratories, Taplow, Maidenhead, Berks SL6 0PH   (Gold Cup SMA)

Xotic, Unit 2, Meadow Lane, Alfreton, Derbyshire   (Nekton additives; Livefoods—mealworms, buffalo worms, crickets, locusts, wax moths, fruitflies etc.)

GLOSSARY

ALTRICIAL NESTLING Immature when hatched and entirely dependent on parental feeding (the Latin *altrix* means feeder or nurse); *see also NIDICOLOUS*

AMPHIBIAN A vertebrate class within the animal kingdom including species which live both on land and in water and have moist, scaleless skins (toads, frogs, newts)

AVICULTURE The breeding of birds in captivity

CARNIVORE Meat-eater. The carnivorous order of mammals includes cat family, dog family, mustelids, seals

CAROTID ARTERY Main artery, supplying blood from heart to head

CETACEAN Member of an order of completely aquatic mammals (whales, dolphins, porpoises)

CHELONIAN Member of order of shelled reptiles (tortoises and turtles)

CHICK Down-covered young of gamebirds and waterfowl, able to run about within hours of hatching. Some are able to find their own food. *See also PRECOCIAL* and *NIDIFUGOUS*

CLASS A grouping within the hierarchical scientific classification system, which divides living organisms into the following increasingly smaller sections:

KINGDOM (ANIMAL or PLANT)

PHYLUM (for animals: VERTEBRATE or INVERTEBRATE)

CLASS (within the vertebrates: MAMMALS, BIRDS, FISH, AMPHIBIANS, REPTILES)

ORDER (subdivision of a CLASS, e.g. CARNIVORE, PRIMATE, FALCONIFORMES or day-hunting birds of prey, GALLIFORMES or gamebirds)

FAMILY (group of similar organisms within a CLASS, e.g. *Canidae* or dog family, *Felidae* or cat family)

GENUS (plural *GENERA;* subdivision of a FAMILY, with a name forming the first part of a Latin term for a particular organism and given a capital letter, e.g. *Homo, Canis, Mustela*)

SPECIES (plural *SPECIES;* the smallest grouping within the usual classification system, identifying a group whose members have the greatest mutual resemblance, e.g. *Canis familiaris* is the domestic dog, and *Canis lupus* is the common wolf. The species is denoted by the second word in the Latin name. A member of a species will breed successfully only with another of the same species in normal circumstances.)

CORVID Member of the crow family (including magpies and jays)

CRUSTACEAN Member of a class of arthropod invertebrates, often with a hardened cuticle "shell", e.g. crabs, shrimps

FLEDGLING Young bird of a nidicolous species which has grown enough feathers to be able to fly and therefore leave the nest, though it will remain dependent on parental help for finding its food for a while

GLOTTIS Opening of the windpipe

GRANIVOROUS Grain and seed eater

HACKING BACK Falconry term for training and exercising a captive hawk to be able to return to the wild—the method is also sometimes used in rehabilitating captive owls

HARDBILL Bird which is capable of feeding by cracking seeds

HERBIVORE Plant-eater

INSECTIVORE Insect-eater. Amongst the mammals, the insectivore order includes the hedgehog, the mole and the shrews

LAGOMORPH Member of the order which includes rabbits and hare

MAMMAL Member of the vertebrate class Mammalia—and in this country in the sub-class Placentalia (in which the young develop within the uterus). Mammals produce milk for their young and have hair; the class includes the great majority of non-bird animals in this book, i.e. carnivores, insectivores, rodents, lagomorphs, bats (*Chiroptera*), ungulates, cetaceans and pinnipedes

MUSTELID Member of a large family of small carnivorous mammals with prominent scent glands, often pungent. Most have long, slender bodies and short legs. Sub-families include *Mustelidae* (marten, polecat, ferret, mink, stoat, weasel); *Melinae* (badger); *Lutrinae* (otter)—all with "locking" jaws

NESTLING Young dependent bird, hatched naked and still without adequate feathering to leave the nest; entirely dependent on parental feeding

NIDICOLOUS Birds which are relatively undeveloped at hatching (lack of feathering, for example) and stay in the nest for some time after hatching, dependent on parents

NIDIFUGOUS Birds which are well developed at hatching, covered with down and able to run: they leave the nest within hours of hatching and many are able to feed themselves

OMNIVORE Animal willing and able to consume wide variety of foodstuffs, whether of animal or plant origin

PASSERINE Member of the order of perching birds (three toes forwards and one backwards)—includes most of our familiar garden birds and song-birds but not water birds, birds of prey, gamebirds and sea birds

PINNIPEDE Member of a mammalian order of specialised aquatic carnivores, including seals and walruses

PISCIVORE Fish-eater

PRECOCIAL Young bird or mammal partially independent at birth, that is, not blind, naked and helpless

PRIMARY FEATHERS Bird's main flight feathers

RAIL Member of a bird family including coots and moorhens

RAPTOR Bird of prey, with sharp talons and strong hooked beak. Birds of prey include the diurnal (daytime) raptors—hawks, falcons and eagles—and the largely nocturnal owls, though the term is commonly applied only to the diurnal raptors. All have forward-facing eyes, which is typical of any predatory animal

REPTILE Member of a class of cold-blooded, egg-laying vertebrates, including snakes, lizards, tortoises and turtles

RODENT Member of a mammalian order with continually growing teeth for gnawing. Includes rats, mice, dormice, voles and squirrels

SCOURING Diarrhoea in young animals

SOFTBILL Bird which feeds on softer foods such as insects and fruit

TRACHEA Windpipe

UNGULATE Member of the order of hoofed mammals, which is divided into the odd-toed (*Perissodactyla*) including horse, mule and donkey, and the even-toed (*Artiodactyla*) including cattle, pigs, sheep, goats and deer

BIBLIOGRAPHY

Anderson-Brown, A.F., *The Incubation Book* (Saiga, 1979)
Association of British Wild Animal Keepers, *The Hand-Rearing of Wild Animals* (ABWAK, 1988 Symposium), *Management of Canids and Mustelids* (ABWAK, 1980 Symposium)
Beebee, Trevor, *Frogs and Toads* (Whittet, 1985)
Beer, J.V., *Diseases of Gamebirds and Wildfowl* (Game Conservancy, 1988)
Brice, Ian, *Barn Owls: Some Aspects of Multibreeding Captive-Bred Barn Owls* (POP)
British Herpetological Society, *The Care and Breeding of Captive Reptiles* (BHS)
Coles, B.H., *Avian Medicine and Surgery* (Blackwell Scientific, 1985)
Cooper, Jo, *Hand-Feeding Baby Birds* (TFH Inc., New Jersey, 1979)
Cooper, John E., and Eley, J.T. (eds): *First Aid and Care of Wild Birds* (David & Charles, 1979)
Cooper, John E. (ed.), et al., *Manual of Exotic Pets* (BSAVA, revised 1985)
Cooper, Margaret E., *An Introduction to Animal Law* (Academic Press, 1987)
Corbet, G.B., and Southern, H.N., *The Handbook of British Mammals* (Blackwell, 2nd edition, 1977)
Ferris, Chris, *Out of the Darkness* (Unwin Hyman, 1989)
Flegg, Jim, *Birdlife* (Pelham, 1986)
Forestry Commission, *Wildlife Ranger's Handbook* (FC, 1985)
Fowler, M.E., *Zoo and Wild Animal Medicine* (W.B. Saunders, Philadelphia, 1986)
Garfield, Rorke, *Animal First Aid* (NARA, 1981)
Godfrey, G., and Crowcroft, P., *The Life of the Mole* (Museum Press, 1960)
Harris, Stephen, *Urban Foxes* (Whittet, 1986)
Heath, J.S. (ed.), *Aids to Nursing Small Animals and Birds* (Bailliere Tindall, 1978)
Holm, Jessica, *Squirrels* (Whittet, 1987)
Jordan, W.J., and Hughes, John, *Care of the Wild* (Macdonald, 1982)
Lawrence, M.J., and Brown, R.W., *Mammals of Britain: Their Tracks, Trails and Signs* (Blandford, 1967)
Lint, Kenton C. and Alice Marie, *Feeding Cage Birds* (Blandford, 1988), *Diets for Birds in Captivity* (Blandford, 1981)
Low, Rosemary, *Hand-Rearing Parrots and Other Birds* (Blandford, 1987)
Macdonald, David, *Running with the Fox* (Unwin Hyman, 1987)
Macdonald, David (ed.), *The Encyclopaedia of Mammals* (George Allen and Unwin, 1984)
McBride, Anne, *Rabbits and Hares* (Whittet, 1988)
McKeever, U.S., *Care and Rehabilitation of Injured Owls*
Mark Martin, Richard, *First Aid and Care of Wildlife* (David & Charles, 1984)
Mead, Chris, *Owls* (Whittet, 1987)
Meaden, Frank, *A Manual of European Bird-Keeping* (Blandford, 1979)
Mellanby, K., *The Mole* (Collins, 1971)
Meyer, Richard, *The Fate of the Badger* (Batsford, 1986)
Neal, Ernest, *The Badger* (Collins, 1948)
Parkes, Charlie, and Thornley, John, *Fair Game: The Law of Country Sports and the Protection of Wildlife* (Pelham, 1988)
Parry-Jones, Jemima, *Falconry—Care, Captive Breeding and Conservation* (David & Charles, 1988)
Pemberton, John E. (ed.), *Birdwatcher's Year Book* (Buckingham Press, annual)
Porter, Val, and Brown, Nicholas, *The Complete Book of Ferrets* (Pelham, 1985)
Pringle, Alan J. (ed.), *Papers of the First Owl Symposium* (1987)
Ratcliffe, Jane, *Fly High, Run Free* (Cicerone Press)
Richardson, Phil, *Bats* (Whittet, 1985)
Ridgway, S.H. (ed.), *Mammals of the Sea: Biology and Medicine* (Charles C. Thomas, 1972)
Robbins, Charles T., *Wildlife Feeding and Nutrition* (Academic Press, New York, 1983)

Shawyer, Colin, *The Barn Owl in the British Isles* (Hawk Trust, 1987)
Stocker, Les, *The Complete Hedgehog* (Chatto & Windus, 1987), *We Save Wildlife* (Whittet, 1986)
Thompson, Arthur R., *Nature by Night* (Ivor Nicholson & Watson, 1931)
Thompson, H.V., and Worden, A.N., *The Rabbit* (Collins, 1956)
Universities Federation for Animal Welfare,
    Humane Killing of Animals (UFAW, 4th edition, 1989).
    The Management and Welfare of Farm Animals (UFAW, 1988),
    Humane Control of Land Mammals and Birds (UFAW, 1984 Symposium),
    The Welfare and Management of Wild Animals in Captivity (UFAW, 1972 Symposium)
Wayre, P., *The Private Life of the Otter* (Batsford, 1979), *The River People* (Collins & Harvill, 1976)
West, Geoffrey (ed.), *Black's Veterinary Dictionary* (A. & C. Black, 16th edition, 1988)

Also numerous free publications by RSPCA, especially: *First Aid for Stranded Crustaceans, Orphaned Foxes*

PERIODICALS

The Aquarist, Buckley Press, The Butts, Half Acre, Brentford.
Cage & Aviary Birds, Surrey House, 1 Throwley Way, Sutton SM1 4QQ.
Feathered World, Winkley Publishing, Preston, Lancs.
The Fox, Fox Press, Oak Tree, Main Road, Colden Common, Winchester, Hants.
Fur and Feather, Winkley Publishing.
Racing Pigeon Pictorial, 19 Doughty Street, London WC1N 2PT.
Ratel, ABWAK members' bimonthly.

INDEX